Promoting the Development of Young Children with Cerebral Palsy

A Guide for Mid-Level Rehabilitation Workers

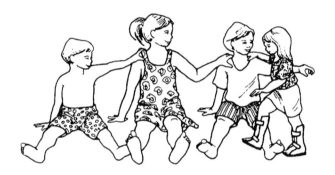

World Health Organization
Geneva
1993

World Confederation for
Physical Therapy

World Federation of
Occupational Therapists

Abstract

This manual is for mid-level rehabilitation workers to use when they work with children who have cerebral palsy and their families, and with other rehabilitation or health workers. The manual includes information on early detection of cerebral palsy and assessment of the level of development of the child. Training suggestions are given for promoting mobility, self help and communication skills. Splints and equipment are shown which can be locally made and used for the prevention of deformities. Some adaptations may be needed for use in specific countries.

CONTENTS

Foreword   iii

1. Introduction

What is Cerebral Palsy ?	1
About This Guide	2

2. About the Condition

Types of Cerebral Palsy	3
Questions Families Ask About Cerebral Palsy	5
Problems Found with Cerebral Palsy	7
Prevention of Cerebral Palsy	9

3. Recognising the Condition

Normal Development	11
How To Use the Development Charts	11
Development Charts	12
Early Signs of Cerebral Palsy	15

4. Planning Training

Principles of Training	17
Assessment and Progress Form	18
General Goals of Training	20
Working Effectively With the Child and His Family	21
Guidelines for Teaching Parents and Families	22

5. Communication

What Is Communication ?	23
Communication and Cerebral Palsy	23
Principles of Training	23
Training Suggestions	24
Alternative Ways of Communicating	26

6. Good Handling	Lifting and Carrying	29
	Handling	30
	Handling the Head	30
	Handling the Body	31
	Handling the Arms and Hands	32
	Handling the Legs	33
7. Preventing Deformities	Good Positions	35
	Positioning in Lying	35
	Positioning in Sitting	36
	Positioning in Standing	39
	Contractures and Deformities	40
	Prevention of Contractures	41
	How to Stretch Muscles Passively	42
	Splints	43
	Assessment and Treatment of Contractures	44
8. Training Suggestions	About the Training Suggestions	47
	Stage One	49
	Stage Two	55
	Stage Three	63
	Stage Four	71
9. Taking Account of the Problems Found With Cerebral Palsy		75
	Children with Severe Difficulties	76
10. Summary of When to Ask for More Help		77
11. Further Reading		79

FOREWORD

This manual has been prepared in response to a need expressed within community based rehabilitation programmes for a text on cerebral palsy which can be used by mid-level rehabilitation workers (MLRWs)*. The manual can be used by teachers for training MLRWs, and by the MLRWs as a reference for their work.

The need for this manual was expressed despite the extensive range of texts devoted exclusively or in part to treatment procedures for children with cerebral palsy. After consultation with representatives of the World Confederation of Physical Therapy (WCPT) and the World Federation of Occupational Therapists (WFOT), we concluded that there was not a text on cerebral palsy appropriate for use by MLRWs. Therefore, we collaborated with WCPT and WFOT in the preparation of this manual.

We wish to express our gratitude to the two individuals who prepared the text: Ms Liz Carrington, selected by WCPT, and Mr Michael Curtin, selected by WFOT. These two authors prepared a draft, which was sent out for review to physical and occupational therapists in each of the six World Health Organization Regions. The therapists selected for the review were individuals with experience working both with children who have cerebral palsy and with MLRWs. Their enthusiastic response to the draft, and their thoughtful comments, were also appreciated. Based on those comments, the completed text of the manual was prepared by the authors. We also wish to thank Ms Shona Grant, who prepared all of the illustrations.

Dr Enrico Pupulin
Chief Medical Officer
Rehabilitation Unit
World Health Organization
Geneva
Switzerland

* Countries have different titles for MLRWs, e.g., rehabilitation assistants or technicians, or physical or occupational therapy assistants.

1. INTRODUCTION

What is Cerebral Palsy ?

Cerebral palsy is a condition that disables children. It is a disorder of muscle control that causes difficulty with moving and positioning the body. A small part of the brain that controls movement has been damaged early in life before or after birth, whilst the child was still a baby. The muscles receive the wrong instructions from the damaged part of the brain. This makes them feel stiff or floppy. The muscles are not paralysed.

Sometimes the damage affects other parts of the brain, which may cause difficulty with seeing, hearing, communicating and learning.

Cerebral palsy affects children for life. The damage to the brain does not get worse, but as the child gets older the effects become more noticeable. For example, deformities can develop.

Cerebral palsy affects each child differently. A mildly affected child will learn to walk with slightly unsteady balance. Other children may have difficulty with using their hands. A severely affected child may need help learning to sit and may not be independent in daily tasks.

Cerebral palsy is found in every country and in all types of families. About one in every three hundred babies born will have, or will develop cerebral palsy.

All children with cerebral palsy can benefit from early teaching and training to help them with their development. Although there is no cure, the effects can be reduced depending on how soon we start to help the child and how damaged the brain is. The earlier help is started, the more improvement can be made.

About this guide

This Guide will help Mid-Level Rehabilitation Workers (MLRW) to assist community rehabilitation workers and families who will train young children with cerebral palsy. It gives information on how to identify young children who may have cerebral palsy and to know when to ask for help from a therapist or doctor. The MLRW can also teach others, such as Primary Health Care Workers (PHCW), how to identify these children in the community.

It gives information about the condition which all rehabilitation workers and families need to know to be able to identify problems and plan activities which will help the child to function better. Training suggestions are given to help the child grow and develop in the best possible way.

The Guide explains how to practise these in the daily routine of the family, for example when washing or playing with the child.

Together, rehabilitation workers and families can encourage the child to move, communicate, play and learn to become as independent as possible.

This Guide should be translated into the language used by the rehabilitation workers and families. Changes may be needed to make it more suitable in a particular community. For example equipment shown in the Guide might be different from things already used in a community to help children move.

Put drawings of your local equipment in the translated version of the Guide.

Throughout this Guide reference will be made to specific Training Packages which come from "Training in the Community for People with Disabilities", World Health Organisation, 1989 (see reference on page 79). These Training Packages will provide more information on some of the topics discussed in this Guide. However, these Training Packages do not contain information specific to cerebral palsy which is why this Guide has been produced.

Using this Guide and the selected Training Packages will help rehabilitation workers and families when training children who have cerebral palsy.

2. ABOUT THE CONDITION

Types of Cerebral Palsy

Spastic Spastic means stiff or tight muscles. The muscle stiffness makes movement slow and awkward. Wrong instructions from the damaged part of the brain cause the body to be held in typical abnormal positions that the child finds hard to move out of. This causes a lack of variety of movements. Gradually deformities can develop.

Muscle stiffness is worse when he is upset, using a lot of effort, or being moved too quickly. Shifts in stiffness from one part of the body to another can occur with changes in the head position.

Spastic cerebral palsy is the most common type of cerebral palsy.

A spastic child is described according to which parts of his body are affected.

<u>Hemiplegia</u>

Arm, body and leg affected on one side.

<u>Diplegia</u>

Legs affected more than arms.

<u>Quadriplegia</u>

Whole body affected.

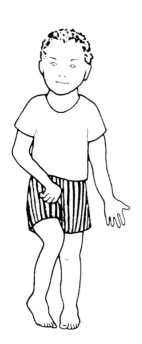

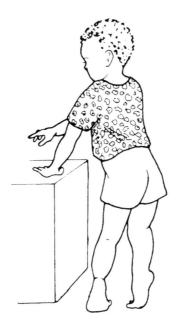

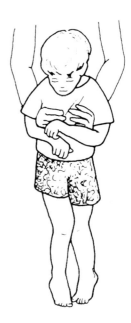

Arm turned in and bent.
Hand fisted.
Leg turned in and bent.
Tiptoe standing.

Arms slightly clumsy.
Legs pressed together
and turned in.
Tiptoe standing.

Poor head control.
Arms turned in and bent.
Hands fisted.
Legs pressed together and
turned in.
Tiptoe standing.

3

Athetoid   Athetosis means uncontrolled movements. These are jerky, or slow wriggly movements of the child's legs, arms, hands or face. The movements occur most of the time. They get worse when the child is excited or upset and much less when she is calm.

Abnormal body positions come and go as the muscles change from stiff to floppy. Deformities are less likely to develop. This constant change makes it difficult to keep still, so balance is poor. If the face is affected, it may be harder to talk clearly enough to be understood.

Athetoid children are **floppy as babies**. They usually develop uncontrolled movements at two to three years of age. This happens gradually. A few children **remain floppy**.

Ataxic   Ataxia means unsteady shaky movements. These unsteady movements are seen only when she tries to balance, walk or do something with her hands. For example when a child reaches for a toy she may miss the first time.

Standing and walking take longer to learn, because balance is poor.

Mixed   Many children show features of more than one type of cerebral palsy. For example, some children have spastic cerebral palsy with athetoid movements.

Athetoid

Ataxic

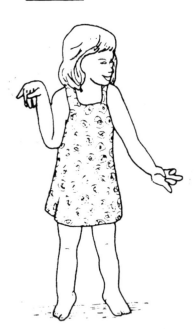

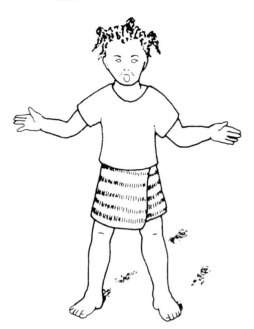

Jerky, or slow wriggly movements of her legs, arms, hands and face. Poor balance.

Unsteady shaky movements. Unsteady walking. Poor balance.

Questions Families Ask About Cerebral Palsy

This information is to help rehabilitation workers answer the questions parents often ask.

What causes it ?

Before birth

. Infection in the mother in the early weeks of pregnancy, for example German measles (rubella) or shingles.

. Uncontrolled diabetes and high blood pressure in the mother during pregnancy.

Around the time of birth

. Damage to the brain in babies born before nine months.

. Difficult birth which causes injury to the head of the baby.

. The baby fails to breathe properly.

. The baby develops jaundice.

After birth

. Brain infections such as meningitis.

. Accidents causing head injuries.

. Very high fever, due to infection or water loss from diarrhoea (dehydration).

In many cases the cause is not known.

Can it be prevented ?

Not entirely, whichever country you live in. It is possible to reduce the numbers of children likely to get it by making sure that pregnant women go for regular health checks (see page 9).

Is it infectious ?

No. No one else will catch cerebral palsy from a child who has it.

Will it happen again ?

It is very unusual for two children in one family to be affected.

Will medicines help ?

Not usually, unless the child has fits (see page 8).

Will an operation help ?

Operations cannot cure cerebral palsy. Sometimes they are used to correct contractures (muscles which have shortened) or to weaken the pull of spastic muscles to prevent contractures developing. But they may make the movement difficulty worse. Only children who are already walking are usually considered for an operation. The best way to help young children is to prevent contractures developing by encouraging active movement in good positions which stretch the tight muscles (see Sections 6 and 7).

Will my child walk ?

Everyone is anxious about this but the answer becomes clear only as the child gets older. Many children with cerebral palsy do not start to walk until they are seven years or older. Less severely affected children will start earlier.

Standing balance must develop before the child is ready to walk.

Children who stand stiffly on tiptoes when held, are not ready to walk. Their jerky steps are due to a baby movement called reflex stepping, which must disappear before proper walking can develop.

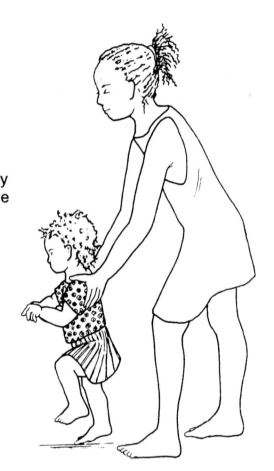

Not all children will learn to walk.

It is important to concentrate on other areas of development. Learning to eat, wash, dress, play and communicate will allow them to join in with family life.

Problems Found With Cerebral Palsy

Eyesight

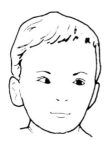

The most common problem is squint. Many young babies do squint from time to time but this stops as they get older. Children older than six months, with a squint, should be taken to an eye doctor because neglecting it can mean that the child only uses one eye.

A few children may need an operation. Others will be helped by wearing glasses prescribed by an eye doctor.

See "WHO Training Packages 1 and 2"

Hearing

Some children, especially those with athetoid cerebral palsy, may have damaged hearing. This makes learning to speak more difficult. If you think he has a hearing problem, consult a doctor. Some children can be helped with a hearing aid.

See "WHO Training Packages 4 and 5"

Eating and speaking

Eating and speaking both depend on the ability to control the muscles of the tongue, lips and throat. When muscle control is poor, there may be difficulties with learning to chew and swallow. Learning to speak can be delayed. Helping a child to eat more normally is an important preparation for learning to speak. Make sure he has enough to eat. Try to feed him some solid food so he can learn to chew.

With encouragement and opportunity most children with cerebral palsy learn to speak but sometimes the words are not clear enough for other people to understand. When this is so, needs may have to be expressed in other ways, such as pointing (see Section 5).

Growth

Babies with eating difficulties may be slow to gain weight. Older children may be thinner than usual because they move about less and do not develop their muscles. In children with hemiplegia, the affected arm and leg are usually thinner and shorter than the other arm and leg.

Slow to learn

Children who cannot talk clearly or control their faces very well are often thought to be mentally slow. This is not always so. About half the children with cerebral palsy have difficulty with learning. Others, especially those with athetoid cerebral palsy, have average or good intelligence.

Personality and behaviour

Cerebral palsy can affect the development of the child's personality. Because he has difficulty moving and communicating, he may become more easily frustrated or angry when doing something, or he may just give up and not try. It is important to always be patient and encouraging and to try to understand him.

Fits (epilepsy)

Fits can start at any age but not all children are affected. Uncontrolled fits may damage the brain further and lower the child's ability to learn. Fits can usually be controlled with medicine, so it is important to consult a doctor.

Medicine may need to be taken regularly for several years and should not be stopped without the advice of a doctor.

Mild fits: The child may stop what she is doing and stare without blinking. You will not be able to get her attention. There may be some unusual movements. For example, repeated movement of the lips or hands.

Severe fits: If the child is able to stand she will fall to the ground. If she is sitting in a chair she may fall to one side. There will be strong uncontrollable jerking movements of her arms and legs, and loss of consciousness. Saliva will come out of her mouth and her eyes may roll up.

Length of fits: Fits are usually short. Mild ones last only seconds. Severe fits seldom last more than 10 to 15 minutes.

Care of the child who is having a fit: If she is having a severe fit
. Move her away from danger such as fire or sharp objects.
. Loosen tight clothing.
. Turn her onto her side so that saliva can run out of her mouth and breathing is easier (see picture for correct position).
. Stay with her until the fit stops.
. When the fit stops she will be drowsy. Let her sleep.

During a fit DO NOT put anything in the child's mouth.

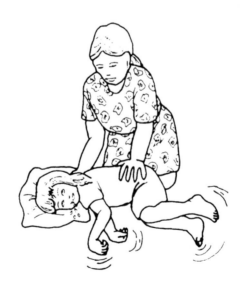

See "WHO Training Package 21"

8

Prevention of Cerebral Palsy

Children will be less likely to have cerebral palsy if these steps are taken:

Before and during pregnancy
. Immunise women against German measles before pregnancy.

. Avoid pregnancy until the woman is 18 years old, and healthy enough to have a baby safely.

. Arrange regular health checks at a health centre. Any problems which might make the birth more difficult can be identified early.

. Check for high blood pressure and ensure treatment if necessary.

. Ensure good nutrition of the woman. This will reduce the risk of premature birth which is an important cause of cerebral palsy.

. Avoid taking unnecessary medicines.

. Arrange the delivery in the safest possible place with a trained person to help.

Care of the baby after birth
. Encourage breast feeding (see page 52). Breast milk protects the baby against infection.

. Encourage regular visits to the health centre so that nutrition, growth and general development of the baby can be checked. Any delay in development can be noticed early and help given (see pages 15 and 16).

. Make sure the baby is immunised against, diphtheria, whooping cough, tetanus, poliomyelitis measles and tuberculosis.

Care of the sick child
. Teach families the early signs of meningitis. These are fever, stiff neck, bulging of the soft spot on top of the baby's head and drowsiness. The child may vomit and may become unconscious. Take the child to a doctor quickly for treatment.

. Teach families what to do if their child has fever. Tell them to keep the child cool, remove his clothes and sponge his body with cool water. Give him plenty to drink. Take him to a health centre for more treatment if the fever does not go down after one full day and one full night.

. Teach families about rehydration for babies with diarrhoea. Tell them to continue breast feeding or giving mashed solid food. Give a glass of rehydration fluid every time the child passes a watery stool. Take him to a health centre if the diarrhoea is not better in two days.

See "The Community Health Worker", WHO, Units 15,16,20 and 21

3. RECOGNISING THE CONDITION

Normal Child Development

An understanding of normal child development helps you to identify children who are not developing as expected, to plan training and to check on progress. Developmental stages are reached in a particular order. The control of the body develops progressively from the head to the feet. Large movements develop before smaller more skilled movements.

The various stages in development, like sitting and standing, are reached at roughly the same age in all children. We decide how well a child is developing by comparing her with other children of the same age. When progress is slower than expected it is called **developmental delay**.

Children with cerebral palsy have a developmental delay. They take longer to learn to control their bodies than other children. Cerebral palsy is just one of a number of conditions which cause delay.

Any child who is not developing as expected should be taken to see a doctor.

How to Use the Development Charts

Although the child with cerebral palsy does not progress in the same way as other children, the stages of normal development are still used as the basis for assessment and training. On the following three pages are the development charts. They differ from the charts found in "WHO Training Package 26", as the charts in this Guide give more detail on the development of movement.

These development charts show the order in which some abilities develop and the age at which most children learn them.

To use the charts: 1. Record the date and the age of the child if known.
                     2. Watch what he can do.
                     3. Tick or circle the things he can do on the charts.
                     4. Try to work out the reasons for a particular difficulty.

This will identify what he can do, what he cannot do, and what he needs to be trained to do.

A child may have abilities spread over two or more stages. For example, a child with diplegia may be in Stage 3 for sitting, Stage 2 for getting to sitting and Stage 1 for standing. This will mean that training suggestions will have to come from all three stages.

DEVELOPMENT CHART: Movement

	Stage 1: Birth to 6 months	Stage 2: 6 to 12 months	Stage 3: 12 to 24 months	Stage 4: 2 to 3 years
Head and Body Control	.Lies on stomach and holds head up .Pushes up on hands / .Rolls from stomach to back	.Rolls from back to stomach .Rolls to side and gets into sitting		
Sitting	.Sits only with support / .Sits leaning on hands	.Sits alone .Twists and reaches / .Catches self if pushed	.Moves into and out of sitting / .Balances self if tilted	
Moving from Place to Place	.Stands with support	.May crawl or shuffle on bottom / .Pulls to stand	.Walks alone or with one hand held / .Squats to play	.Kicks a ball / .Balances on one foot .Jumps

12

DEVELOPMENT CHART: Communication and Behaviour

	Stage 1: Birth to 6 months	Stage 2: 6 to 12 months	Stage 3: 12 to 24 months	Stage 4: 2 to 3 years
Using Hands	.Holds small object briefly .Holds with whole hand	.Can hold one object in each hand	.Holds between thumb and finger	
Playing and Social Development	.Looks at object .Brings hands together .Plays with body .Hits object with whole arm	.Plays social games like peek-a-boo .Passes object from hand to hand .Bangs two objects together	.Puts objects into container and takes them out .Enjoys building	.Throws a ball .Sorts different objects

DEVELOPMENT CHART: Communication and Behaviour

Self-Care

Stage 1: Birth to 6 months	Stage 2: 6 to 12 months	Stage 3: 12 to 24 months	Stage 4: 2 to 3 years
.Sucks breast .Takes object to mouth	.Chews solid food .Feeds self biscuit	.Drinks from a cup and feeds self most foods without help .Helps with undressing .Indicates toilet needs	.Dresses with help .Uses the latrine without help

Communication

Stage 1: Birth to 6 months	Stage 2: 6 to 12 months	Stage 3: 12 to 24 months	Stage 4: 2 to 3 years
.Responds to noises .Makes sounds when talked to .Smiles .Turns to voices Hello · Ah ah · Shathani · Na na	.Likes being talked and sung to. .Repeats gestures .Repeats sounds made by others .Responds to simple commands .Says a few words "Ma ma", "Da da", "Ba ba" Bye bye · Ball	.Calls self by name .Names familiar things like dog, bird .Uses a lot of nonsense talk .Asks for things with words and gestures .Begins to put words together .Points to body parts when asked Drink · Where is your nose?	.Talks about what she does .Begins to draw .Asks questions .Helps family members with their work

14

Early Signs of Cerebral Palsy

The early signs of stiffness or floppiness may be noticeable soon after birth. Other signs may take several months before they become obvious. **To be sure that the child has cerebral palsy, take him to a doctor.**

The following signs are of concern if they are seen most of the time. Not every child will show all of these signs.

Things Families Notice

. <u>Sudden stiffening</u>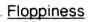

In some positions, like lying on the back,
it becomes difficult to bend the baby's body,
to dress or cuddle him.

. <u>Floppiness</u>

The baby's head flops and he cannot lift it.
His arms and legs hang down when he is held
in the air.
The baby moves too little.

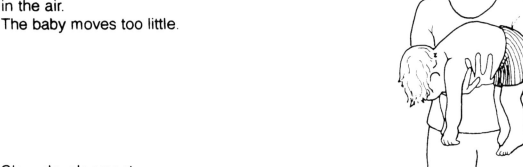

. <u>Slow development</u>

Learning to lift his head, sit and use his
hands takes longer than expected. He
may use one part of his body more than
another. For example, some babies only
use one hand rather than learning
to use both.

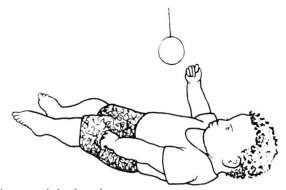

. <u>Poor feeding</u>

Sucking and swallowing is poor. His
tongue pushes the milk and food out.
He has difficulty closing his mouth.

. <u>Unusual behaviour</u>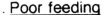

He may be a crying, irritable baby who
sleeps badly. Or he may be a very quiet
baby who sleeps too much. He may not
smile by the age of three months.

More Signs to Look For

The drawings on the left show the way normal babies move at some important stages of development. The drawings on the right show how the same movement might look when done by a child with cerebral palsy. **To be sure that the child has cerebral palsy, see a doctor.**

<u>Age</u>	<u>Normal Development</u>	<u>Cerebral Palsy</u>	

By 3 months

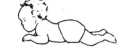 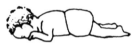 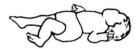

Lies straight on stomach; holds head up well; pushes up on arms.
Lies on back; brings two hands together.

.Stiff legs.
.Cannot lift head.
.Cannot push up on arms.

.Pushes back, head to one side.
.One arm and leg bent, the other arm and leg straight.
.Cannot bring hands together.

By 6 months

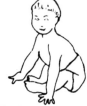 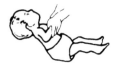

Sits leaning on hands; takes weight on feet when held in standing.

.Cannot lift head.
.Round back.
.Stiff arms and fisted hands.

.Head falls back or pushes back when he is pulled to sitting.

.Tiptoe standing.
.Arms pull back.
.Stiff legs which are crossed like scissors.

By 9 months

Sits alone; reaches out; supports self when placed in standing.

.Round back.
.Poor use of hands for play.
.Stiff legs, pointed toes.

.Does not take weight on legs.
.Poor head lifting.

By 12 months

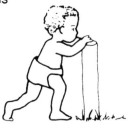 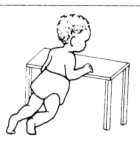 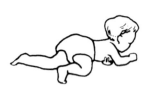

Pulls to stand holding something; crawls well.

.Difficulty pulling to stand.
.Stiff legs, pointed toes.

.Cannot crawl.
.Uses only one side of body or drags self by only using arms.

By 18 months

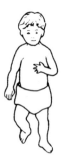 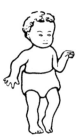 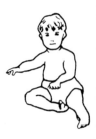

Stands and walks alone; moves into and out of sitting; sits straight; uses both hands.

.One arm stiff and bent.
.Tiptoe walking on one side.
.Poor standing balance

.Uses mostly one hand to play.
.One leg may be stiff.
.Sits with weight to one side.

16

4. PLANNING TRAINING

Principles of Training

Assessment
. Assess the child using the development charts and your knowledge of the different types of cerebral palsy. Take account of the child's personality and behaviour.

. After your assessment, record what he can do, what his needs are and what you plan to do.

. Select training activities according to his needs and the stages of development he has reached.

. Always keep notes on his progress so that training can be changed as he improves (see pages 18 and 19).

Handling and training techniques
. Always talk with the child and his family. Agree on what needs to be done as a priority. Explain what you are doing and why you are doing it. Explain what you want him to do (see pages 21 and 22).

. Give him plenty of time to try to do activities. Reward every effort with praise.

. Use handling techniques to move him into good positions. This makes it easier for him to move himself.

. Provide support when needed but remove it as he does more himself.

. Use equipment only when necessary and only for as long as needed.

. Handling and training should not make unwanted movements worse. A spastic child should not become stiffer. An athetoid child's movements should not become more uncontrollable.

Progress
. Not all children will make the same amount of progress. If the child's progress is poor it may be because:
  - the family are not sure how to train the child.
  - the training activities are too difficult.
  - the family are looking for too much progress too soon.
  - the child is too severely affected to progress quickly.
  - the family are unable to carry out the training.

. When a child is not making progress try one or all of the following:
  - explain the training goals and activities again.
  - point out even very small improvements to the child and family.
  - break activities down into smaller steps.
  - choose easier training activities.
  - ask a therapist for advice on what to expect of the child.
  - assess the family situation and arrange community support if necessary.

Assessment and Progress Form

Always record the child's abilities and difficulties at the first visit and then at regular intervals. This will help you to plan your training programme and to know when to try different training suggestions. Record the equipment supplied.

This is one suggested form on which to record a child's progress. It summarises what has been found when the child is assessed. If you already have a form which fulfils your needs, use it. Remember that no matter which form is used it is important to make notes on a child's progress so that you can see how effective the training suggestions are. This progress form is filled in for a child with spastic right hemiplegia to give an example of how to use it.

ASSESSMENT AND PROGRESS FORM

<u>Name</u>: Lumba M   <u>Date of Birth</u>: November 1991   <u>Age</u>: 18 months
<u>Address</u>: Tsesebe Village   <u>Date of First Visit</u>: 28.5.93
<u>Diagnosis</u>: Not moving right arm and leg   <u>Parts of Body Affected</u>:
normally. Possibly cerebral palsy.

<u>Family Concerns</u> (include early signs): Right arm and leg stiffer to move than the left side. Child has not learnt to use both hands. Does not use right hand. She cannot get into sitting, nor pull up to stand or walk. When held in standing, she cannot keep her right foot flat.

<u>Other Difficulties</u>:   Seeing   (Hearing)   Speaking   Feeling
(circle any problems)

                             Strange   Fits   Learning   Other
                             behaviour   (list them)

<u>Medicine</u>: None taken.

<u>Contractures</u>: None as yet. Range of movements full but resistance to stretching of right knee and foot is moderate and right elbow and hand mild. Has risk of tight right foot.

<u>Summary of Development Chart</u>

Lying on front	Pushes up on left hand only.
Rolling	Rolls to both sides but prefers to roll to the right.
Sitting	Cannot get into sitting. When placed in sitting, balances leaning to the left. Balance only fair - falls when pushed.
Crawling	Does not crawl or bottom shuffle. Moves around by rolling or dragging herself along the floor with her left arm.
Standing	Unable to pull herself up to stand or to walk. Cannot keep her right foot flat when held in standing.
Usings hands and playing	Uses left hand only. Plays with her own body and knows several parts.
Eating	Chews solid food. Feeds herself with the left hand.
Dressing	Only lifts her left arm to help with dressing and undressing.
Speaking	Tries to say words and makes appropriate sounds. Takes an interest in what is happening around her. Does not always turn to sounds.

18

Problem List (In order of priority)	Plan of Action	Date Started	Date Achieved
Not standing. Unable to keep right foot flat. Resistance to stretch moderate.	Practise standing from an adult's knee with help. Discuss ways of doing this during self-care activities to build it into the daily routine.	28.5.93	
	Activities in supported standing to stretch and straighten the leg. If the foot will not press flat, make a plaster of Paris splint.	28.5.93	
Not using right arm. Resistance to stretch mild.	Use activities in sitting and standing which involve pressing down through straight arms. Encourage leaning to the right. Discuss ways of doing this during self-care activities to build it into the daily routine. Teach to hold on with two hands when playing.	28.5.93	
Sitting difficulties.	Do lying to sitting activities. Train sitting balance. Offer toys from the right. Make a chair and tray so she can sit straight. Find a local craftsperson to help with this. Measurements taken. Bring on next visit.	28.5.93

28.5.93 | |

Further Help

Possible hearing difficulty.	Refer to PHCW for hearing test.	29.5.93	
Diagnosis.	Refer to doctor to confirm diagnosis.	29.5.93	

Equipment Supplied	Chair and tray. Plaster of Paris footsplint.		

Next Visit: 9th July 1993.

General Goals of Training for All Types of Children with Cerebral Palsy

Spastic Child

. Relax stiff muscles.
. Encourage movements which avoid spastic body positions.
. Prevent deformities.

Floppy Child

. Provide support in a good position.
. Encourage movements so that the muscles become stronger.

Athetoid Child

. Learn to hold on with hands to steady uncontrolled movements.
. If abnormal body positions come and go, also follow the goals for a spastic child.

Ataxic Child

. Improve balance in kneeling, standing and walking.
. Stand and walk steadily.
. Control unsteady shaky movements, especially of the hands.

For All Children With Cerebral Palsy

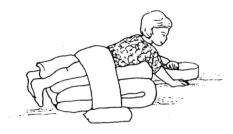 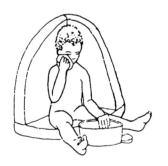 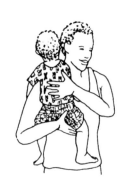

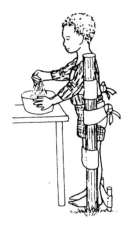

. Encourage movement in as normal a way as possible.
. Use both sides of the body.
. Follow the developmental stages.
. Encourage child to learn by doing activities related to daily life.
. Position the child straight in lying, sitting, kneeling and standing.
. Prevent deformities.

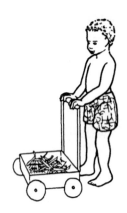

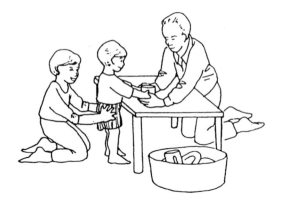 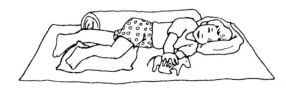

20

Working Effectively With the Child and His Family

All children need to be talked and listened to. They need to be played with and praised and rewarded for the things they learn to do. This helps them to develop.

A child with cerebral palsy takes longer to learn to do things. For example, he may be slow to smile or reach out. This may make his family take less notice of him. They may not reward him for any progress he makes. Because he does not get rewarded, he may stop trying and this will further delay his development.

Some families overprotect their child who has cerebral palsy. They do too much for him. He will not learn to do things for himself. Other families want to teach their child to do things before he is ready. This may make abnormal movements worse. The rehabilitation worker can help families know where to start with their child. It is best to start with activities that he can already do. Build on his success and follow the stages of development (see pages 12 , 13 and 14).

Families and rehabilitation workers need to learn from one another. The family will know their child best. For example, if he has difficulty talking, a member of his family can help the rehabilitation worker to understand him. The rehabilitation worker can suggest ways to make the daily care of the child easier for the family.

Rehabilitation workers should:

. Listen to the family and observe the child in different situations. For example, when he is eating or being washed or dressed.

. Notice what he can already do.

. Agree on which problem is most important.

. Respect and encourage helpful things the family are already doing with their child.

. Praise the child for what he can do and for attempting to do things, however small.

. Make training suggestions practical and relevant to family life.

. Make training fun for the child so that he will want to do the activities.

. Make sure you do not give the family more to do than they have time for.

. Show all the members of the family how to help, so that they all can be involved with training the child.

Guidelines for Teaching Parents and Families

. Show and explain the activity you are teaching.

. Guide and encourage the members of the family in doing it.

. Show how the activity can be practised in daily life.

. Answer any questions the family have about the activity.

. Leave some instructions.

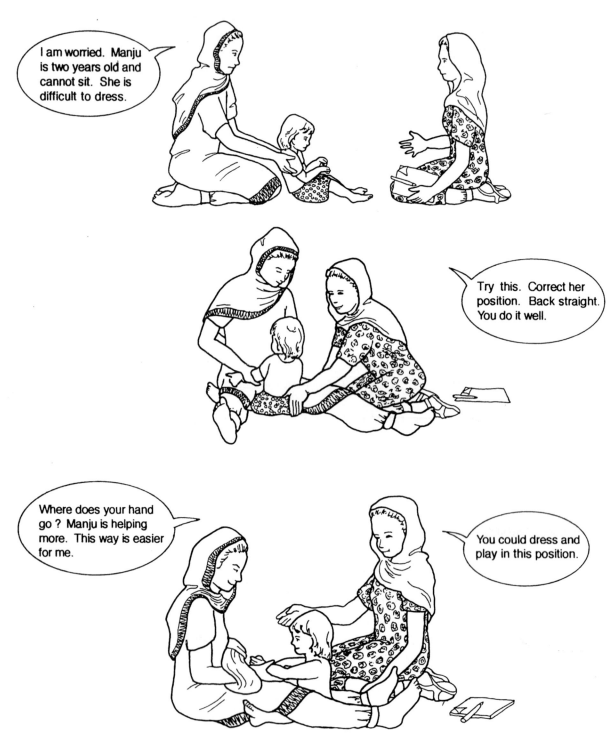

22

5. COMMUNICATION

What is Communication ?

Communication is the way in which we understand messages from other people and the way in which we express our thoughts, needs and feelings to them.

Children who can hear, communicate mostly through spoken words.
Other ways to communicate include:
. Voice - crying, whining, laughing.
. Body movement, for example nodding the head.
. Facial expressions such as smiling.
. Gestures such as waving goodbye.
. Pointing with the eyes or the finger.
. Writing and drawing.

Communication and Cerebral Palsy

Most children with cerebral palsy can hear, so they listen to the words you say and in time begin to use words themselves. Listening and understanding comes **before** talking.

Children who have difficulty controlling movements of the head, face, mouth and tongue will have difficulty in saying words clearly. If other people do not understand when the child tries to speak he may become frustrated and stop trying.

It is important to encourage him to communicate in any way possible. Teach the family to notice all the ways in which he is communicating.

Principles of Training

. Position the child to relax his body. Sitting is a useful position in which to learn to speak.
. Help the child to sit straight and to keep his head upright so he can concentrate on looking and listening.
. Encourage eating and drinking in a good position as a preparation for speaking (see pages 7, 52, 59, and 66).
. Face the child. Talk to the child at his eye level so he can see you and can keep his head forward. Get his attention.
. Use single words or simple short sentences when you speak to the child. Use gestures with words to help him to understand more of what you say.
. Give him time to respond.
. Accept all the methods of communication which the child uses and praise him for his efforts so he will keep on trying.
. Encourage the family to give the child the opportunity to communicate. Give him choices such as "Do you want water or juice ?" Wait for him to point or try to reply.
. Give the child a means of attracting your attention. If he cannot call you, give him a bell to hit or a rattle to shake.
. Use alternative methods of communication if he finds speaking difficult after several months of training (see page 26).

Training Suggestions

Stage 1

The child begins to take an interest in her surroundings but does not understand words. She learns that she can affect what other people do. For example when she cries, some one will come. She communicates by using facial expression and sounds.

Call her name. When she looks at you praise her by smiling and talking. Use lots of facial expression.

When she makes a sound, copy it and then take turns at talking.

Talk to her about everyday sounds and what they mean. For example, footsteps mean someone is coming, the clatter of pots means meal time.

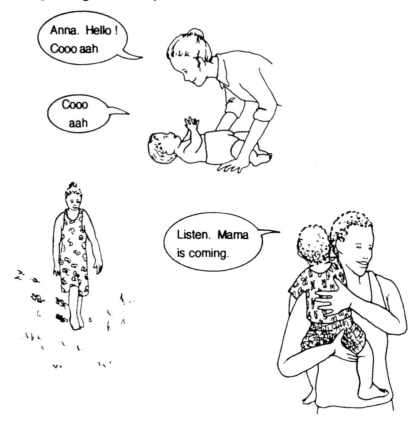

Stage 2

Although she does not use words of her own, she understands and copies a few words other people say. She understands gestures. She communicates by using her own gestures and a variety of sounds which are similar to words.

Let her play with everyday objects that make different sounds. Let her watch you working. Talk about what you are doing. Sing songs to the child. She will enjoy the rhythm.

Ask the child to do simple things. Use gestures as you speak. For example, "Give me your hand", "Wave bye bye" or "Hold the ball". Wait for her to move.

Try to understand what she means when she uses sounds. Help her to use them as words. If she says "Ba" when playing with a ball, say "Yes, there is your ball".

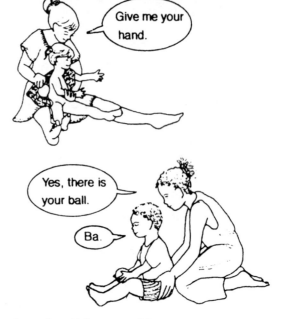

Do not try to correct her way of saying things at this stage.

24

Stage 3

The child says single words. He uses particular sounds and gestures which carry meaning.

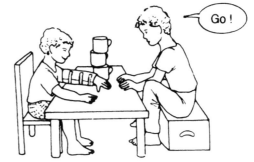

Build a tower. Show him how to knock it down. Build it again. Make him wait for you to say "Go" before he knocks it down again.

When washing and dressing, name his body parts and clothes. Play "Show me your nose", "Show me your foot".

Give him a choice of things to play with and to eat. Show him the choices, well spaced out, where he can see them best. Ask him "Do you want water or milk ?" "Do you want the ball or the doll ?" Notice how he indicates, by word, sound, finger or eye pointing.

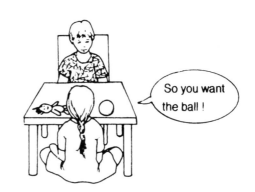

Stage 4

The child uses simple two or three word sentences to give information and to ask questions.

Tell the child stories and ask him questions about them. encourage him to point to pictures and to name people and things. Answer his questions.

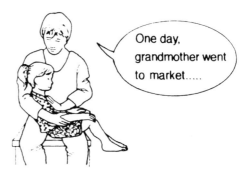

Help him to put two words together. Use words he knows in games and everyday situations. For example "My turn", "Hello Maria", "More rice", "Shirt on".

Talk about where people and things are.
"I am **next** to you".
"The ball is **on** the table".

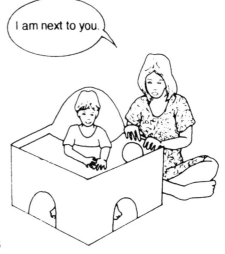

Listen to him when he tells you what he is doing. The words the child uses may still not be very clear to people who do not know him well. At this stage, children begin to get frustrated if they cannot make themselves understood.
If the child tries for several months to say new words but cannot do so, try another method of communication.

Alternative Ways of Communicating

If the child is having difficulty learning to speak, encourage her to use other ways of communicating her thoughts, needs and feelings. Notice whether she is already using other ways, such as pointing to things with her finger or her eyes. Or she may use a special movement of her head or hands to say things.

Make sure the family rewards her for **all** the ways in which she tries to communicate. As she becomes more successful at making her needs understood, she will want to communicate more and may begin to use words.

Asking Questions   If you are sure the child is understanding you, try to develop a consistent "Yes", "No" signal. If she has difficulty learning to speak, encourage her to use one sound or movement for "Yes" and another sound or movement for "No". For example she might blink her eyes for "Yes" and raise her hand for "No".

If she can communicate with a "Yes" and "No" consistently, alternative communication methods can develop. Find out what she wants to do or to have by asking "Yes", "No" questions such as "Do you want a drink ?"

Picture Boards   If the child cannot use her hands well enough to use sign language but she can indicate "Yes", "No", try a picture board. Collect pictures from newspapers or calendars which show things that the child and her family do. Stick a few really useful pictures onto a piece of stiff card or a wooden board. Make them into a book if the child is using a lot of pictures.

Examples of pictures

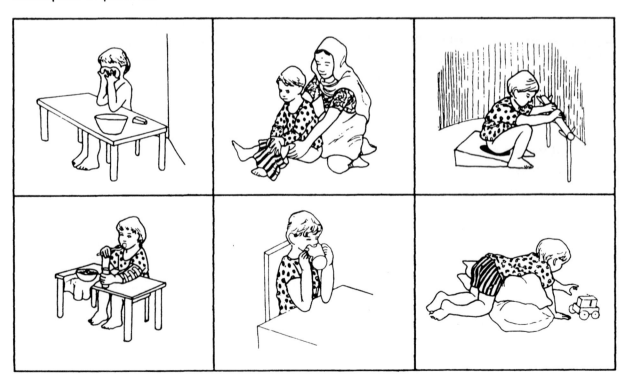

Pointing to Pictures

Position the child so he can relax and concentrate on pointing. Make sure he can see the pictures. Explain the pictures to the child. Ask him to point to the picture of what he wants to have or to do. Give him what he asked for in the pictures.

Problem Solving

. If the child is able to move his arm to touch the pictures but cannot open his hand, then let him use his fist to point. Make sure the pictures are well spaced out on the board.

. If the child cannot reach the pictures because he holds his elbow bent, then use a gaiter splint to keep his elbow straight (see page 43).

. If the child cannot use his arm or hand to point, then point for him. Encourage him to use a sound or movement to tell you when you are pointing to a picture of something he wants, or see if he can point with his eyes by looking at the picture of what he wants.

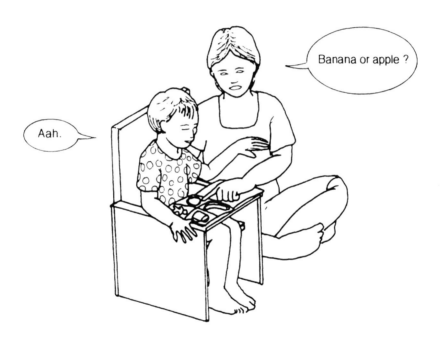

Sign Language	Some children with cerebral palsy will have enough control over their hand movements to be able to use sign language. If there is a set of signs in use in your country for people who have difficulty hearing and speaking, let the child try them.
	The child who has difficulty moving her hands may make up her own signs. Make sure everyone who knows the child understands her signs.

See "WHO Training Package 7"

6. GOOD HANDLING

Lifting and Carrying

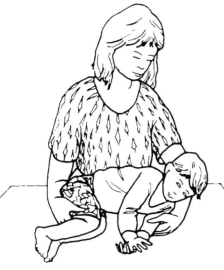

Lifting
To make it easier to lift the child and to prevent abnormal positions:
. Roll him to one side and support his head.
. Bend his legs.
. Lift him close to your body.
. Put him down the same way.

Carrying
Carry him in a way which corrects abnormal positions and which brings both his arms forward. A more upright position helps him learn to hold his head up and look around.

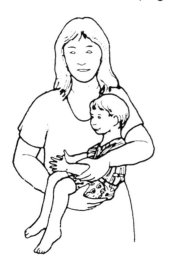

All very young children can be carried like this.

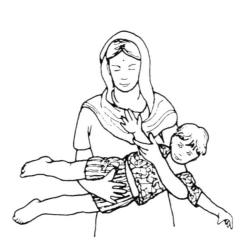

A good position to straighten a spastic child.

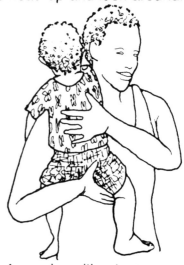

A good position to carry a spastic child whose legs cross, or a floppy child.

A good position to carry a spastic child whose legs cross, or an athetoid child.
Use this for short distances.
You can swing him from side to side in this position.

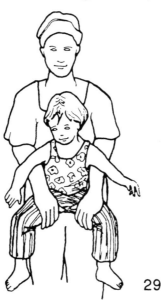

A child can be carried on your back. If he needs more support or his head is floppy, carry him on your side.

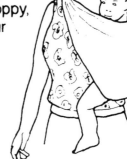

Handling

Handling is a way of supporting and guiding a child so that her movements become more normal.

Good handling relaxes a stiff child. It supports a floppy or athetoid child. It allows ataxic and athetoid children to control their movements more.

**Good handling is the basis of ALL the training suggestions.
It makes it easier to care for your child.**

Handling the Head

<u>Handling To Avoid</u>

<u>Handling To Encourage</u>

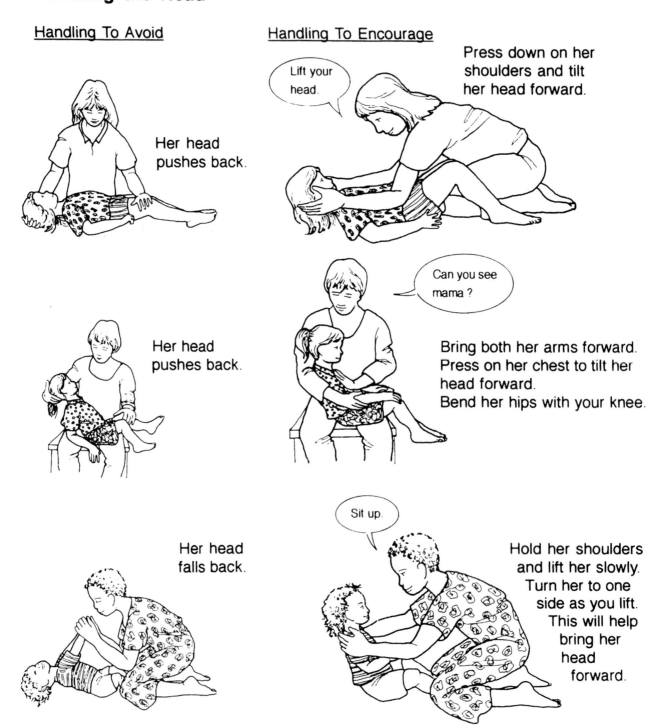

Her head pushes back.

Lift your head.

Press down on her shoulders and tilt her head forward.

Her head pushes back.

Can you see mama?

Bring both her arms forward. Press on her chest to tilt her head forward. Bend her hips with your knee.

Her head falls back.

Sit up.

Hold her shoulders and lift her slowly. Turn her to one side as you lift. This will help bring her head forward.

Handling the Body

Handling To Avoid Handling To Encourage

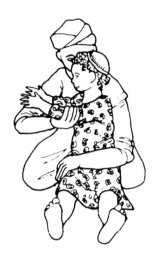

To relax a spastic child:
. Twist his body from
  side to side.
. Twisting can also be
  done in lying (see
  page 50).
.For a bigger child,
  straighten his knees
  by putting your legs
  over them.

A floppy child's
sitting position.

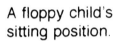

Yes, your ball.

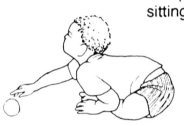

Baw.

To straighten the back:
. Hold him around his
  hips.
. Press down.

If he is very floppy:
  . Support his chest
    with one hand.
  . Press down on his
    lower back with
    your other hand.

Sit still. Look.

When sitting
unsupported
an athetoid
child's arm
and leg
movements
may be
uncontrolled.
His body may
push backward.

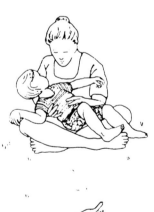

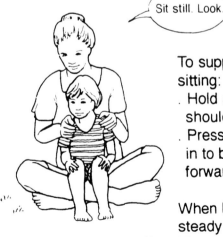

To support him in
sitting:
. Hold around his
  shoulders.
. Press them down and
  in to bring the arms
  forward.

When his sitting is
steady it is easier for
him to look
and listen.

31

Handling The Arms and Hands

<u>Handling To Avoid</u>   <u>Handling To Encourage</u>

A spastic child's arms may be bent and pulled back. Her hands may be closed.

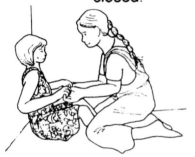

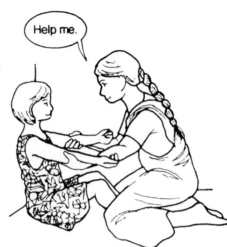

To straighten her arms:
. Hold around her elbows.
. Turn the arms out as you bring her forward.

If the arms are difficult to bend:
. Hold her around the elbows.
. Turn her arms in.

If her muscles are spastic, never pull the fingers and thumb out by their tips. This will make the hand close more tightly.

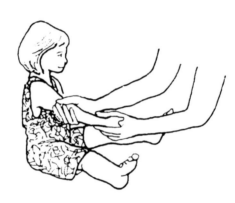

To open her hand:
. First straighten her arm
. Hold her hand so her thumb is away from the palm
. Bend her wrist back while gently opening the hand.

To lean on her hands:
. Straighten her arms as above.
. Bend one wrist back while gently opening the hand.
. Place the palm flat on the ground.
. Do the same for the other hand.

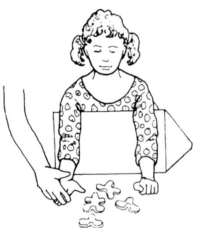

<u>To help her to hold things</u>
see pages 66 and 70.

<u>Other ideas to open the hand</u>
. Shake her arm rhythmically while supporting the shoulder and elbow.
. Stroke the back of the hand on the side of her little finger. When the hand is open, rub her palm with different materials, such as wool, cotton and sheepskin. She will get used to touching different things.

Handling the Legs

<u>Handling To Avoid</u>

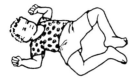

A floppy child may lie with his legs apart.

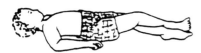

A spastic child's body will be straight and his legs will press together or be crossed when lying on his back.

If the muscles are spastic, never pull the legs apart. This will make the legs pull together more.

<u>Handling To Encourage</u>

To bring them together see page 35.

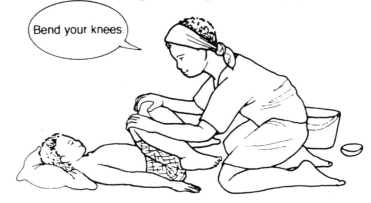

Bend your knees.

To part his legs:
. Put something under his head and shoulders to hold them forward.
. Hold his knees.
. Bend his legs up.
. As his hips bend the legs will part.

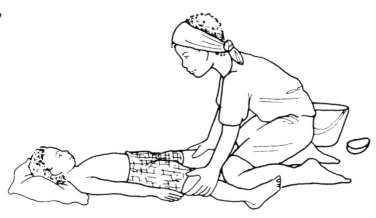

Then:
. Hold him around the knees.
. Keep his legs apart as you straighten them.
This may help his feet to bend up more easily.

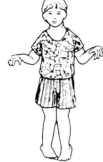

He may stand on the insides of his feet with his knees together.

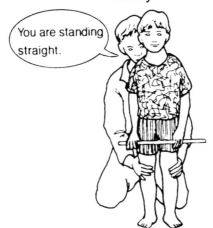

You are standing straight.

To stand with his feet flat:
. Hold around the knees .
. Turn both knees out.

Holding a stick with both hands will give him more control of his arms while standing.

7. PREVENTING DEFORMITIES

Good Positions

A good position enables a child to do more for himself in a normal way. Allow him some movement rather than fixing him completely with equipment. Too much support does not allow him to learn to move. Change his position regularly.

Positioning in Lying

Choose the position which corrects your child best:

Lying on his front

. Place him on a roll, wedge or cushion.

. This keeps his arms forward and helps him to lift his head.

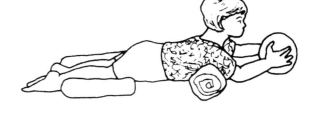

. Hold floppy legs together with cushions or sandbags.

. Hold stiff legs apart with a roll.

. Straighten bent hips with two sandbags joined with a strip of material.

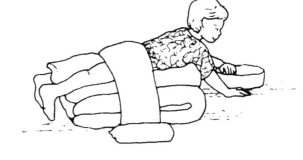

Side lying

. Keep both arms forward to bring his hands together.

. Bend one hip and knee. This stops his legs from pressing together and relaxes his body.

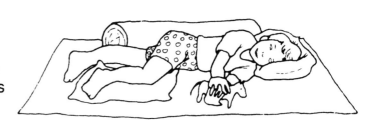

Lying on his back

. Bring his head and shoulders forward.

. Bend his hips and knees. This prevents his body from becoming stiff and straight.

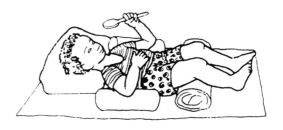

Positioning in Sitting

The child with delayed sitting will need more support. She will require this support for a longer time than other children. She may need a special chair to help her to sit in a good position so she can use her hands better and chew and swallow more easily. The child who is learning to sit, should also practise standing activities.

Good sitting

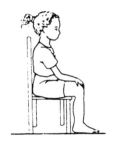

. Head slightly forwards.
. Back straight, no leaning to one side.
. Bottom level against the back of the chair.

. Knees over feet.
. Legs slightly apart.
. Feet flat on the floor or supported by a footrest.

Positions to discourage

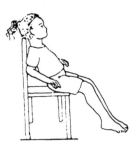 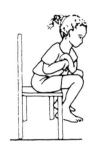

. Hips too straight.
. She pushes back and slides out of the chair.

. Hips too bent.
. She falls forward.

How to measure for a chair

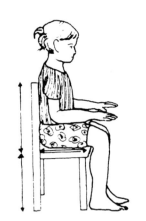 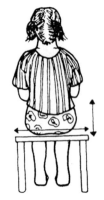

Seat back height - armpit to bottom.

Seat height - back of knee to heel.

Chair arm height - seat to elbow.

Seat depth - back of bottom to back of knee, less width of two fingers.

Seat width - width of bottom plus width of two fingers.

Problem solving

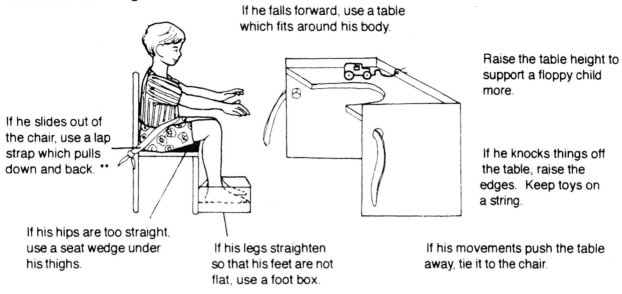

If he falls forward, use a table which fits around his body.

Raise the table height to support a floppy child more.

If he slides out of the chair, use a lap strap which pulls down and back. **

If he knocks things off the table, raise the edges. Keep toys on a string.

If his hips are too straight, use a seat wedge under his thighs.

If his legs straighten so that his feet are not flat, use a foot box.

If his movements push the table away, tie it to the chair.

** If uncontrollable movements are strong, a groin strap may be better (see page 38). Pad the straps. Check that the child does not get sore skin.

Problem solving

If the child's legs press together use a sit astride seat. This chair is cut out of a cardboard box.

Sit the child astride a roll of cardboard, or a filled sack, covered with a towel.

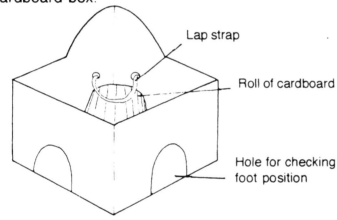

Lap strap

Roll of cardboard

Hole for checking foot position

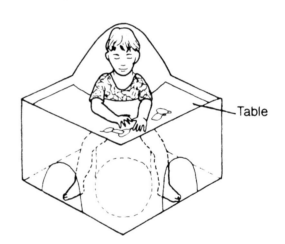

Table

How to Make the Seat

Close the flaps at one end of the box and glue them shut. Stand the box on this end. Cut it into two pieces to make the chair and table.

Cut the table to fit around the child's body.

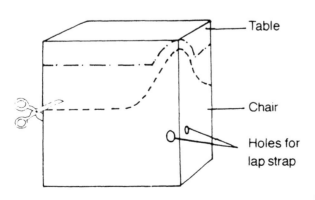

Table

Chair

Holes for lap strap

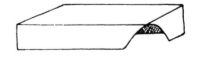

If he needs a stronger chair, glue three layers of cardboard together and strengthen the edges with brown paper. Varnish the chair to make it waterproof.

Problem Solving

If the child's knee bending muscles are in danger of shortening sit her with her legs straight. If she needs support use a corner seat. Also encourage standing.

This chair can be made from wood, foam or cardboard.

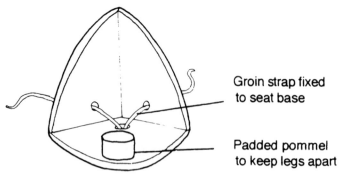

Groin strap fixed to seat base

Padded pommel to keep legs apart

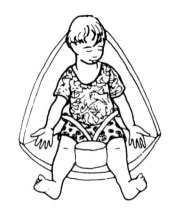

How to Make the Seat

Foam: Use firm thick foam. Glue the pieces together. Strengthen the chair by gluing it into the corner of a cardboard box. Trim the edges of the box to fit.

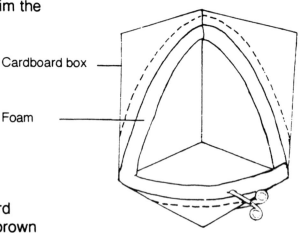

Cardboard box

Foam

Cardboard: Glue three layers of cardboard together. Strengthen the edges with brown paper. Varnish the chair to make it waterproof.

Problem Solving

If she pushes back, add a base to stop the chair tipping.

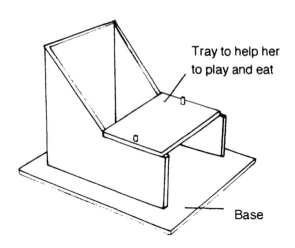

Tray to help her to play and eat

Base

If she cannot sit with a straight back and straight knees (even with knee gaiters), raise the chair off the floor so the knees can bend (see page 73).

Positioning in Standing

Children with delayed standing can benefit from standing supported in a good position. Standing encourages the muscles that hold the body up to work. It prevents contractures and strengthens leg bones. The child has his hands free for play, can see more and can communicate more easily with others.

Good standing

Body in a straight line and feet flat with equal weight on both of them. Hips are straight.

Problem solving

If he needs support to stand and his body is bent, or he cannot keep his heels on the ground, use a forward lean stander.

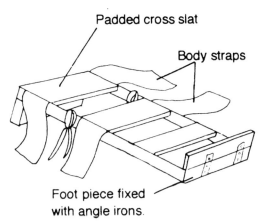

Padded cross slat

Body straps

Foot piece fixed with angle irons.

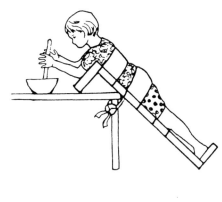

If he needs less body support use an upright stander. Make sure the upright poles are pushed well into the ground or fix them to a large square base for use indoors.

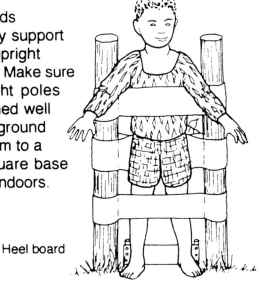

Heel board

For children who lean back, bring the chest strap right around the body. Tie at the back.

Pull the ends of the bottom strap firmly to straighten the hips. Tie the ends securely over the bottom.

Ways to correct and straighten the feet

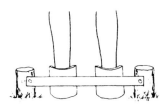

The feet turn out.

Use wedges, foam or buried bricks to correct the feet.

Use cardboard heel cups made from three layers glued together, or a piece of plastic drainpipe to keep the feet straight.

Contractures and Deformities

A **contracture** is a shortened muscle which prevents the full range of movement being carried out at a joint. The joint becomes stiff.

A **deformity** is an abnormal position of a joint. Eventually the joint may not move at all.

Causes

Too little movement

When the child is floppy she moves less than usual and stays in one position.

Muscle imbalance

This happens when some muscles are stronger than others. For example the spastic child is pulled into abnormal positions by overactive spastic muscles.

Assessment

Watch her moving

Which positions does she use most ? Are these positions to encourage or discourage ? Are any muscles in danger of shortening ?

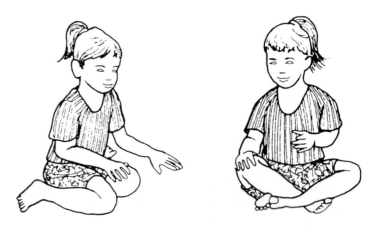

For example, this child **always** sits with her legs bent. The muscles which bend the hips and knees will shorten. Then standing will be difficult.

These positions are only bad if they are used all the time. Encourage other sitting positions too, such as sitting on a low stool.

Check range of movement at each joint

Which muscles already feel tight because of contractures ? Will the muscles stretch ? How far will they stretch (range of motion) ? How easy or difficult are they to stretch (resistance to stretch) ?
Record what you find using the method you have been taught.

Plan action

Prevention of Contractures

. **Use correct handling and positioning** to help relax spastic muscles (see pages 29 to 33).

. Encourage **active movements** (the child moves himself) into or within good positions, which will stretch tight muscles. Make this part of his daily life (see pages 47 to 74).

For example dressing like this will stretch bent hips:

. If resistance to stretch is increasing, the tight muscles will need to be held in a position which gives a **constant stretch** over longer periods of time. This will be more effective. Use a **positioning aid** (see pages 35 to 39, and 76) or a splint (see page 43). Choose positions which will be helpful for the child in daily life. For example, a standing frame will straighten the child's bent legs but also free his hands for play. He should not be left in one position for too long or he will become stiff and uncomfortable. When he is not using any equipment, encourage a variety of active movements.

. Add daily **passive stretching** (you move the child) for muscles which are most in danger of shortening and for existing contractures. This will keep the range of movements as full as possible. Also use it while splints are being made for him. Passive stretching alone will not be enough to prevent contractures. Use the other methods first.

Progress

Keep a check on the range of movement of his joints. If the contracture is still getting worse and the resistance to stretch is increasing, take the child to a physical or occupational therapist, or a doctor. Plasters or braces may be needed to correct the contracture. It should not be necessary for young children to have surgery to correct contractures (see page 6). **Now is the time to work hard on preventing contractures**.

Summary of Assessment and Action

Assessment of Resistance to Muscle Stretch	Assessment of Range of Joint Movement	Action
Mild	Full	Use good positioning and handling. Encourage active movements into or within good positions.
Moderate	Full	Add a constant stretch using a positioning aid or splint.
Strong	Limited - contracture starting.	Add daily passive stretching.
Very strong	Decreasing - contracture still getting worse	Take him to see a therapist or a doctor. He may need plasters or braces to correct the contracture.

How To Stretch Muscles Passively

. Explain what you want to do. Get the child's co-operation first.

. Position the child so as to reduce any stiffness or abnormal movements (see pages 35 to 39).

. Hold the limb in a stretched position. **Stretch very slowly and gently** as you count to 20.

. As the muscles relax, stretch them a little more.

. Repeat the stretching and counting for 5 minutes. Do this twice a day. Once in the morning and once in the evening.

For example, when stretching the foot:

Support her leg behind her knee.

Pull down on the heel rather than bending the foot up, to protect the joints of the foot.

As you stretch, do not allow the heel to tilt to one side.

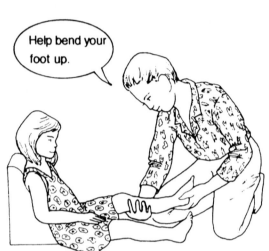

Help bend your foot up.

Some muscles lie over two joints. For example, the calf muscles cross the back of the knee and the ankle. If the muscles are tight, stretching one joint will cause the stiffness to shift to the other. Straightening the knee may make it more difficult to bring the heel down. So it is best to straighten the knee and pull the heel down **at the same time**, so the muscles are fully stretched. This will help her to stand correctly with both feet flat on the ground.

Things to be careful about

. Do not cause any pain or fear by using force. **Stretch very slowly and gently**.

. Do not move joints to and fro with a pumping action. This gives a quick stretch which increases stiffness in spastic muscles. Wait for the child's body to adapt to the stretch.

. Do not stretch during sudden stiffening or uncontrollable involuntary movements. Wait for the muscles to relax first.

. Be careful not to overstretch the joints. Never stretch floppy muscles.

. Practise stretching when doing self-care activities.

Splints

Gaiters

These are used to provide a constant stretch to straighten a limb. These lightweight splints are made of strong cloth and reinforced with stiffeners. Stiffeners can be made from strips of metal, plastic or wood. Gaiters wrap around the arm or leg to hold it straight. **Do not** position a stiffener directly over the kneecap or point of the elbow. The straps fasten on the outside of the limb. To begin with try magazines or newspapers wrapped around the limb. If this helps, then make a proper gaiter.

Design of a gaiter   **How to measure for a knee gaiter**

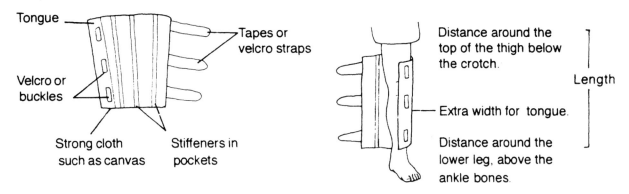

Tongue — Tapes or velcro straps — Velcro or buckles — Strong cloth such as canvas — Stiffeners in pockets

Distance around the top of the thigh below the crotch. — Length — Extra width for tongue. — Distance around the lower leg, above the ankle bones.

How to measure for an elbow gaiter: Measure in a similar way as for the leg gaiter. Measure the distance around the top of the arm, below the armpit, and the distance around the wrist, above the wrist bones. The length is the distance between these two measurements. Use a gaiter if a child is able to straighten the hip and knee, or elbow, with the help it gives. **Do not** use a gaiter if there is a severe contracture. The gaiter will be very uncomfortable and will dig into the leg or arm.

Knee gaiters can be used when lying face down, when sitting on the floor or when standing.
Elbow gaiters can be used to keep one arm forward and still on a table, while the child uses his other arm. They can also be used to help him to bear weight on a straight arm or to help him to reach out and hold on (see pages 72 and 74).

Thumb splint

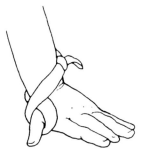

Wind a handkerchief around the base of the thumb to help pull it away from the palm. Tie it on the other side of the wrist. It should not be too tight. This will make it easier for him to hold things or to lean on his hands.

Foot Splints

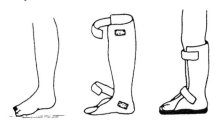

These are used to correct tiptoe standing (see page 65). Use plaster of Paris splints for small children. If stronger splints are needed, see a therapist or doctor. If available, light plastic splints can be worn inside shoes or sandals, or have a rubber sole stuck on the bottom for walking.

Assessment and Treatment of Contractures

If the child is in an abnormal position, first ask her to try and correct it. If she cannot, see how far you can correct it for her. If the tight muscles prevent full correction of the position, there is a contracture.

Will her hips bend and her knees straighten ?

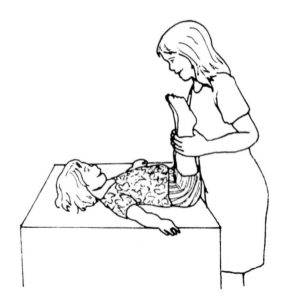

Abnormal position
   . Round back and bent knees.
   . Child leaning back and sitting on the
     base of her spine.

Test position
   . Try to straighten both her back and
     her knees together.
   . Sit her upright on her bottom.

   If this position is not possible there is a
   contracture.

What to do

   . <u>Active movement</u>
   Sitting (see pages 22,51,67 & 70).
   Standing on hands and feet (see pages 63 & 64).
   Standing (see pages 58,63,65 & 71).

   . <u>Positioning</u>
   Sit with straight back and knees.
   Use the wall or a corner seat for back
   support (see pages 38,60 & 73).

   . <u>Constant stretch</u>
   Add knee gaiters in sitting (see page 73).
   If her back is very round in this position,
   sit her on a chair so her knees can bend.
   Encourage standing. Use a standing
   frame or gaiters, depending on how much
   support the child needs (see pages 39 & 74).

   . <u>Passive stretching</u>
   Rest the child's feet against your body.
   Hold her knees and straighten them as far
   as possible.
   Lean forward gently to bend her hips.
   Keep her bottom pressed down flat.

Make all these activities a part of washing, dressing and playing.

Will his hips straighten ?

Abnormal position
> . The child lies with his back arched so his
> feet will touch the floor.
> . He may also stand with his back arched.

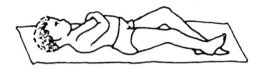

Test position
> . Bend one knee onto his chest to keep his back
> flat.

> If the free leg does not stay flat, there is a hip
> contracture.

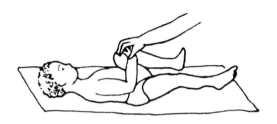

What to do
> . <u>Active movement</u>
> Pull to stand (see pages 58 & 63).
> Walking (see pages 65 & 71).
> . <u>Positioning</u>
> Lying on his front (see page 35).
> . <u>Constant stretch</u>
> Encourage standing in a standing frame (see
> page 39).

Will his legs part ?

Abnormal position
> . The child stands, sits or lies with his legs
> pressed together or crossed.

Test position
> . Part the legs gently (see page 33).

> The dotted lines in the picture show how
> far legs normally part. If they do not part
> like this there is a contracture.

What to do
> . <u>Active movement</u>
> Sitting with parted straight legs (see page 62, 67 & 70).
> Sitting with parted bent legs also (see page 57).
> Side stepping when walking (see page 65).
> . <u>Positioning</u>
> Lying (see page 35).
> . <u>Constant stretch</u>
> Sit astride seat (see page 37).
> Standing frame (see page 39).
> Chair with a knee block (see page 76).
> Side lying board with a leg shelf (see page 76).

Make all these activities a part of washing, dressing and playing.

Will her legs come together ?

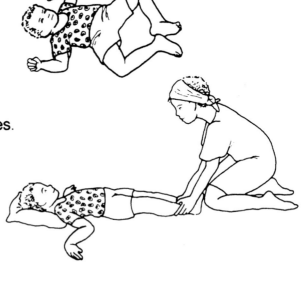

Abnormal position
  . The child lies with her legs apart (usually
   floppy).

Test position
  . Bring her legs together with straight knees.

  If they do not touch there is a contracture.

What to do

  . <u>Active movement</u>
   Kick the legs in lying or sitting in a chair.
  . <u>Positioning</u>
   Keep her legs together in lying or sitting
   with sandbags or cushions (see page 35).
  . <u>Constant stretch</u>
   Use knee gaiters in sitting (see page 73).
   Stand using knee gaiters, or a standing frame,
   depending on how much support is needed
   (see page 39 & 74).

Do her heels stay flat on the floor ?

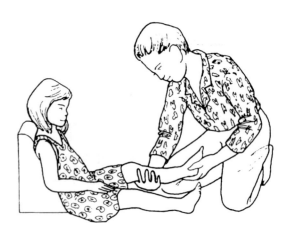

Abnormal position
  . She stands in a tiptoe position (see page 3).

Test position
  . As described on page 42.

  If her heel cannot be brought down so that
  her foot points straight up, there is a
  contracture.

What to do

  . <u>Active movement</u>
   Promote early standing in a good position.
   Train balance for walking (see pages 58, 63 & 65).
  . <u>Constant stretch</u>
   If she still stands on tiptoe, use foot splints (see
   page 43) for standing practise. If she tries to walk on
   tiptoe, continue training balance, but take her to a
   therapist or doctor for advice about splints or braces.
   If available, lightweight plastic splints are often
   helpful (see pages 43, 65 & 71).
   If she requires the support of a standing frame, check
   the position of her feet (see page 39).

Make all these activities a part of washing, dressing and playing.

46

8. TRAINING SUGGESTIONS

About the Training Suggestions

The following are suggestions for training children with cerebral palsy. They are set out in four stages which are the same four stages shown in the Development Charts. Use the Development Charts to see which stage, or stages, a child is at. Then use activities from the same stage and from the next stage, of the training suggestions to train the child. You may be working on several abilities at once. For example, a child who is learning to sit may also need to stand with support.

Some of the self-care activities have to be broken down into smaller steps for the child to practise. Teach the child to do the activity one step at a time. When the child can do one step move onto the next one.

The best way to promote a child's development is to make training activities a part of everyday life. It is important that the activities fit into the child's daily routine.

Explain to the child what you are doing and what you want him to do. Encourage the family to do the same. Encourage the child to help and to talk or communicate with you. Talk with the child, sing songs, tell stories and play games to make doing the activities fun so that the child will want to do them.

Involve all the members of the family if possible. Show them all how to do the activities properly. They all should be aware how to handle the child and how to prevent deformities. Share the responsibility of training. This will be more fun for the child and less strain on one member of the family.

If a child finds it difficult to achieve a goal, check that the activities he is doing are not too difficult. Otherwise, try to achieve the goal using alternative activities. For example, the child who has difficulty lifting his head in lying may be able to do it much more easily in sitting or standing. The child who has difficulty learning to balance his body to sit, may achieve more body balance when standing with support.

The child who has severe cerebral palsy may not progress from one stage to the next. He may show little improvement even after a long time. For him, encouraging communication, good handling and positioning, and preventing deformities are all very important. Equipment may be needed to support him in a good position and so prevent deformities. This will make it easier for his family to look after him.

Finally, these are only suggestions. Encourage the family to think of other things that they can do with their child.

WHO "Training Packages 23 and 26" will provide other information and activities which support the Training Suggestions in this section of the Guide.

STAGE ONE

Stage One: Head and Body Control: <u>Holding the Head</u>

Unless the child learns to lift her head, it will be difficult for other abilities like sitting to develop. Lying on her back can make her press backward and increase body stiffness. Upright positions will help her hold her head up, look around and learn.

Start in supported sitting, because it is easier for her to balance her head in this position.

. Press her shoulders down gently.
. Tilt her backward bit by bit, to teach her to hold her head forward.
. Tilt her further as head holding improves.
. Try tilting slowly from side to side as well.

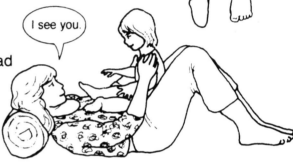

. Give less support as she learns to hold her head forward.
. Move your knees to tilt her from side to side. slowly.

Now train her to lift her head up when she leans forward:

. Lean her forward supported against your body.
. Move her from side to side slowly.

Finally, encourage her to lift her head when lying on her front:

. Support her on your chest.
. Move her from side to side slowly.

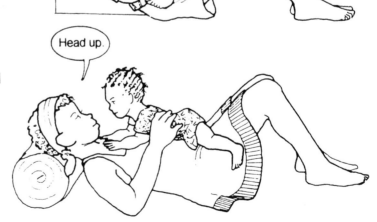

Choose upright positions for feeding, carrying and playing.

Stage One: Head and Body Control: <u>Rolling</u>

Twisting between the upper and lower body is part of normal rolling and is needed later for sitting and walking. When rolling, the head turns to one side, the shoulders follow and then the legs.

Relax his body before training him to roll:

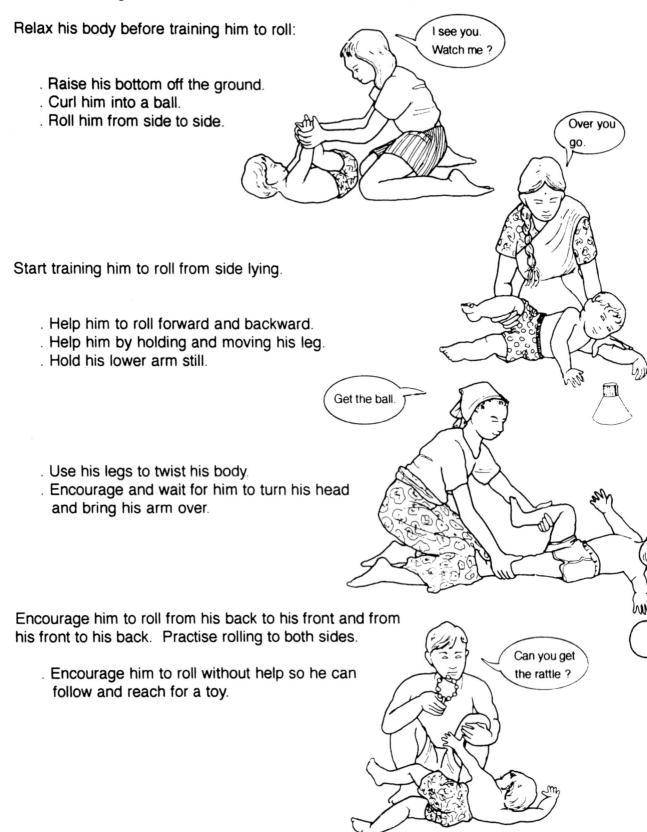

. Raise his bottom off the ground.
. Curl him into a ball.
. Roll him from side to side.

Start training him to roll from side lying.

. Help him to roll forward and backward.
. Help him by holding and moving his leg.
. Hold his lower arm still.

. Use his legs to twist his body.
. Encourage and wait for him to turn his head and bring his arm over.

Encourage him to roll from his back to his front and from his front to his back. Practise rolling to both sides.

. Encourage him to roll without help so he can follow and reach for a toy.

Use rolling when washing, dressing, playing and putting him to sleep.

50

Stage One: Sitting: <u>Sitting Leaning on Hands</u>

Teach the child to hold her body up as she is moved about and to lean on her arms for support. Sitting up will allow her to see both hands and to use them more.

. Keep both her arms forward.
. Twist her body from side to side to touch her feet.
. Lift your knee as you tilt her and encourage body balance.
. Talk to her as you move. Say "Left and right".

. To straighten her back, lift her arms up and forward as you twist her from side to side.

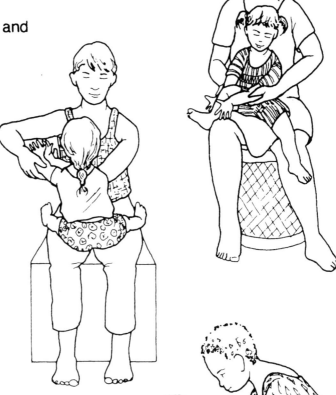

. Hold her hands and feet.
. Tilt her backward and forward, and from side to side slowly to encourage head and body balance.
. Talk to her as you move. Say "Up and down", "Backward and forward".
. Rhythmic words will make the movements fun.

. Hold her knees for support.
. Tilt her forwards so she can catch herself and lean on her arms for support.

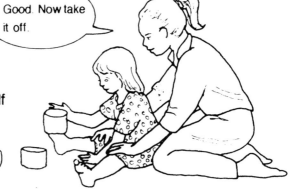

Good. Now take it off.

Also practise sitting on a chair (see pages 36 to 38 and 66).

Sit leaning on hands when washing, dressing and playing.

Stage One: Self Care: <u>Feeding</u>   -   See "WHO Training Package 25"

Helping a child to feed well is an important preparation for learning to speak (see page 7).

Position to Avoid

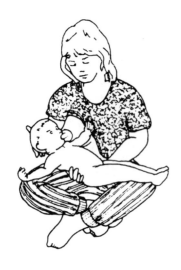

Position to Encourage

Now you can relax and enjoy sucking.

. Child lying flat.
. Head pushing backward.

. Turn his body towards you as much as possible.
. Hold him in a more upright position.
. Keep both his arms forward.
. Press on his chest to tilt his head forward.
. Keep his hips bent over your knee.

This makes sucking and swallowing more difficult.

<u>If he needs more help</u>:

If he is unable to close his mouth, help him by lifting his jaw and pulling his cheeks forward.

If he tends to stiffen backwards, press against his chest with the back of your wrist to tilt his head forward.

This makes sucking and swallowing easier.

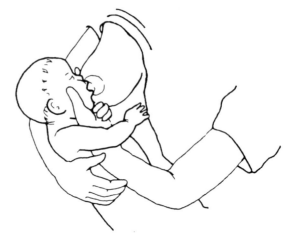

If he cannot suck from the breast or a bottle, use a small spoon to give him milk.

Stage One: Self Care: <u>Washing</u>

Choose the position which controls the child best.

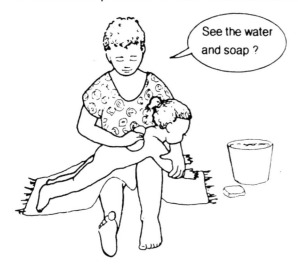

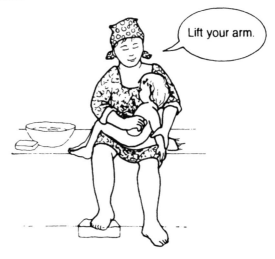

Straighten her hips. Keep her head higher than her hips by lifting your knee up. This will make it easier for her to hold her head up.

Bend her hips by lifting up your knee. This relaxes her body.

Stage One: Self Care: <u>Dressing</u>

Choose the position which controls the child best.

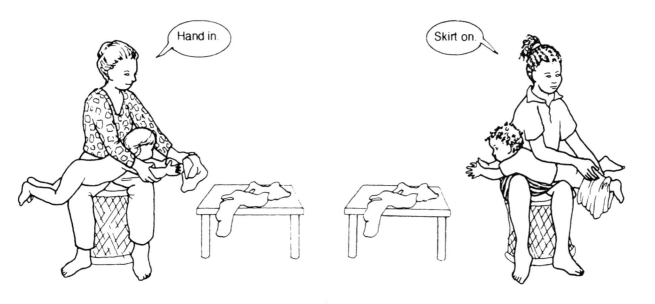

Straighten her hips. Keep her head higher than her hips by lifting your knee. This will make it easier for her to hold her head up.

Dress the most affected side first and undress it last.

**Always place the water and clothes where she can see them.
Tell her what you are doing and talk about her body so she can learn.**

Stage One: Using Hands and Playing

Encourage the child to bring his arms forward and to look at his hands.

Do this in a variety of good positions to help him to practise rolling and sitting.

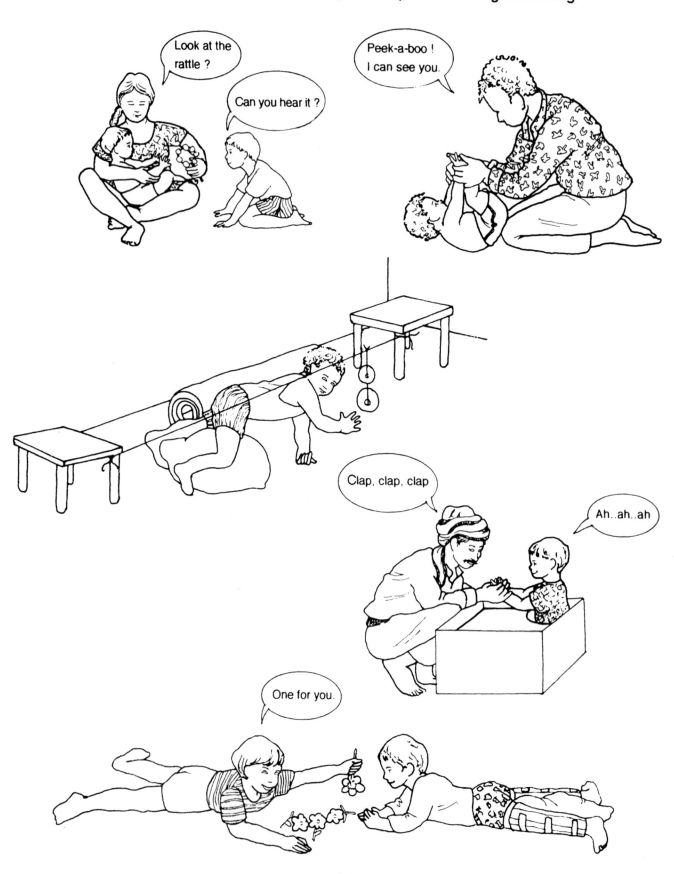

STAGE TWO

Stage Two: Sitting: <u>Preparing for Sitting Alone</u>

Push her forward and sideways so that she learns to catch herself. As the body balance improves she will be able to lift her hands and will not need to lean on them for support. Teach her to twist and reach in all directions.

. Hold her hips.
. Tilt her gently to one side so she catches herself.
. Tilt her to the other side.

Do not fall.

. Sit her to one side.
. Encourage her to reach out in all directions with one hand.
. Hold her other arm straight so she can support herself.

What are you cooking, Kayaga ?

. Lay her over something that rolls, like a bucket or large tin.
. Hold her hips.
. Tilt her slowly forward so she learns to catch herself.

Hands down Nadine.

. Sit her astride your lap.
. Tilt her gently to one side using your knees while supporting her body and encourage her to catch herself.
. To help her sit up, press down on her top hip.
. Tilt her to the other side.

Pick up the leaves.

Children with delayed sitting will also need to use a chair for support (see pages 36 to 38)

Practise sitting when eating, drinking, washing, dressing and playing.

Stage Two: Sitting: <u>Sitting Up From Lying Down</u>

When the child can sit alone, teach him to sit up from lying:

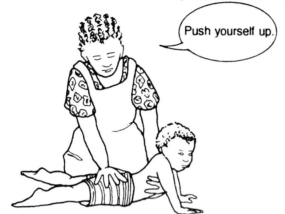
Push yourself up.

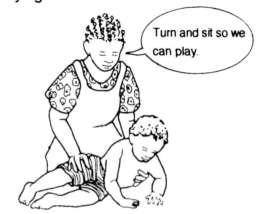
Turn and sit so we can play.

. Support his chest.
. Turn his hips towards you.

. Then press down and back on his hip.
. Support his body as he pushes up on one arm.

When he needs less help, hold his hand as he pushes up.

Practise every time the child needs to sit up to eat, drink, wash and play.

Stage Two: Moving Around: <u>Moving on Hands and Knees</u>

When the child can sit alone teach him to support himself on his hands and knees.
If he crawls with very bent legs, contractures may develop. Instead, encourage him to sit and to stand with straight hips and legs.

Teach him to balance on his hands and knees. This will help him to kneel up and stand.

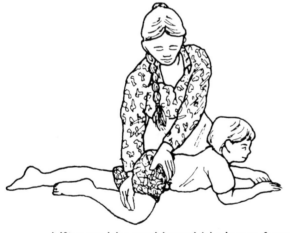

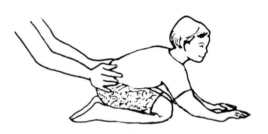

. Lift one hip and bend his knee forward
. Shift his weight onto his forward knee and then bend his other leg in the same way.

Then,
. Press down on both hips to encourage him to lift his head and to support himself on both arms.
. Rock him gently from side to side and backward and forward to train his balance.

If he needs help to get up from the floor, let him get onto his hands and knees before you lift him.

Practise this when washing, dressing and playing.

56

Stage Two: Sitting: <u>Sitting Alone</u>

For good sitting on a chair the child must learn to keep her feet flat on the floor, part her legs, lean forward and hold on with both hands. Praise her when she sits well.

Choose games which keep her in a good position and train balance. Encourage her to keep her elbows straight. If she has difficulty, begin by using elbow gaiters (see page 43).

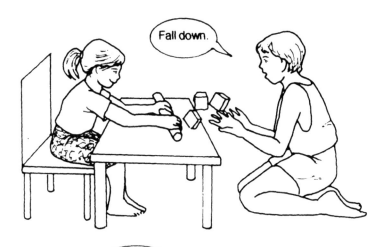

As her balance improves, encourage her to let go with one hand and then with both.

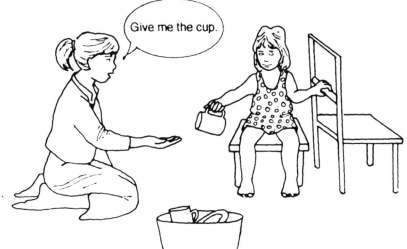

When she no longer needs to hold on, help her to reach in all directions, sitting on a stool. Sing songs with actions for her to copy. Help her to stamp her feet and bend down to touch her toes.

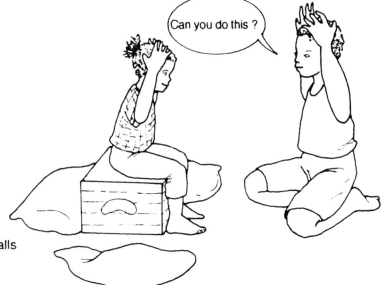

Cushions in case she falls

Practise this when eating, washing, dressing and playing.

Stage Two: Moving Around: <u>Pull to Stand</u>

When pulling to stand children need to lean well forward. Often they push back and this will make standing difficult.

To move from sitting to standing correctly:

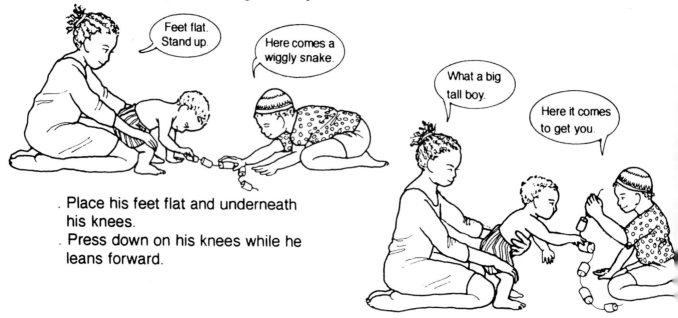

. Place his feet flat and underneath his knees.
. Press down on his knees while he leans forward.

. As he stands, support his chest and knees.

Do not let him lean back.

To move from kneeling to standing:

. Press down on one knee.
. Keep the other knee well back while he leans well forward.
. As he stands support his chest.

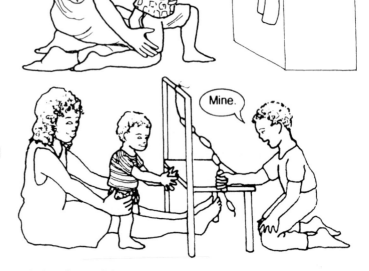

When standing:

. Support him with your leg.
. Hold his hips straight and forward over his feet.
. Shift his weight from side to side.

Many children will need equipment to be able to stand (see page 39). Practise standing when washing, dressing and playing.

Stage Two: Self Care: __Eating and Drinking__

A child can eat or drink on your lap or in a chair. If she needs a lot of support in sitting, and help to chew and swallow, it would be easier to feed her in a chair. Bring her head and arms forward. Always offer food and drink from straight in front, so she can keep her head forward.

When eating:

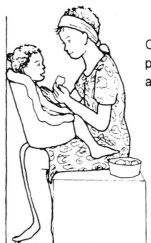

Chair made from plastic bucket and padded.

. Use a spoon for soft foods.
. When using a spoon, place the food on the middle of her tongue.
. Use a shallow spoon which will not break easily.

. To help her to chew, give her small pieces of solid food.
. Place the food to the side of her mouth and toward the back between the teeth.
. If she needs help to keep her mouth closed when she chews, apply firm pressure to her jaw as shown in the pictures below.

When drinking:

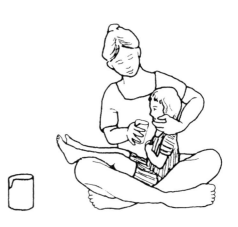

. If she cannot close her mouth apply firm pressure to her jaw as in the pictures below - this will also help with swallowing.
. Cut out a piece of the cup which will fit around her nose - this way she will not have to tilt her head back when drinking.

Controlling the jaw if she is facing you.　　　Controlling the jaw if you sit beside her.

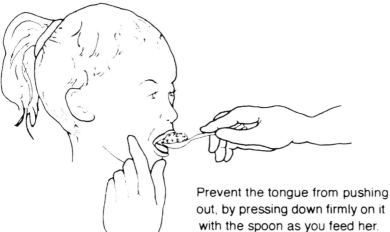

Prevent the tongue from pushing out, by pressing down firmly on it with the spoon as you feed her.

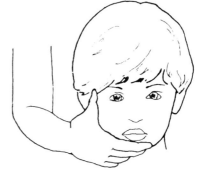

Do not tilt her head backward.

59

Stage Two: Self Care: <u>Washing</u>

Choose a good position to wash the child.

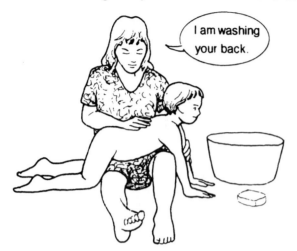

To keep his head higher than his hips, lift your knee. This will make it easier for him to hold his head up.

If he is learning to sit, then wash him in this position.

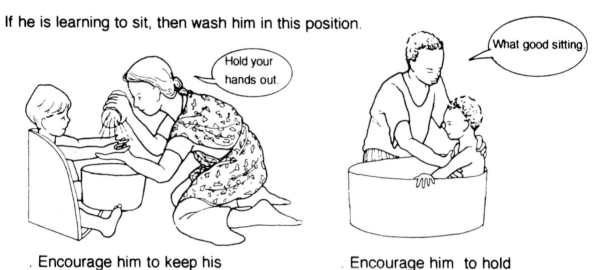

. Encourage him to keep his hands together.

. Encourage him to hold onto the tub.

If he is learning to stand, then wash him in this position.

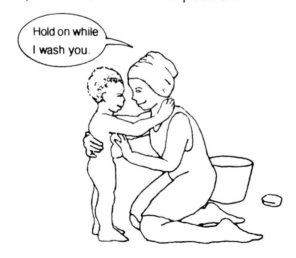

Always place the water where he can see it.
Tell him what you are doing and what you want him to do so he can learn.

Stage Two: Self Care: <u>Dressing</u>

Choose a good position to dress the child.

If she is learning to sit, dress her in this position.

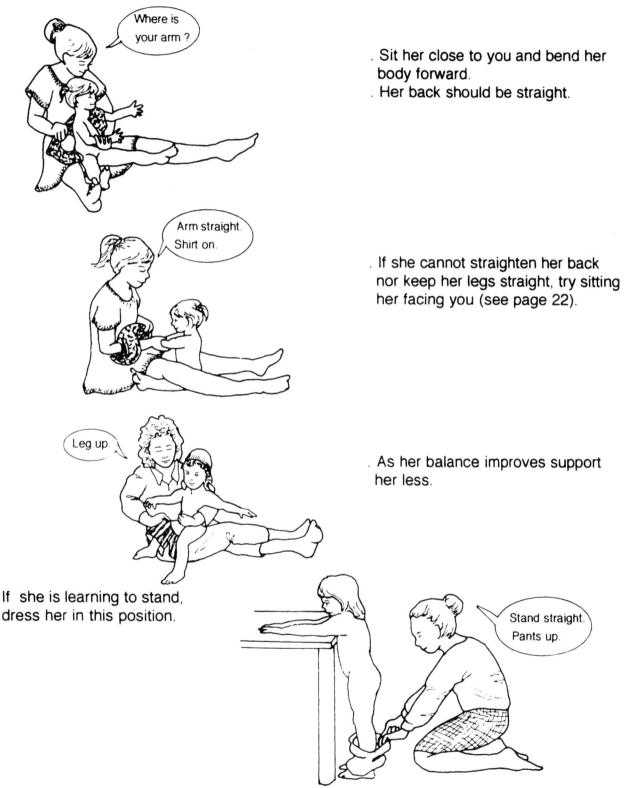

. Sit her close to you and bend her
body forward.
. Her back should be straight.

. If she cannot straighten her back
nor keep her legs straight, try sitting
her facing you (see page 22).

. As her balance improves support
her less.

If she is learning to stand,
dress her in this position.

**Always place her clothes where she can see them.
Tell her what you are doing and what you want her to do so she can learn.
Dress the most affected side first and undress it last.**

Stage Two: Using Hands and Playing

Encourage the child to reach in all directions with both his arms and to lean on his hands.

Do this in a variety of good positions to practise sitting, kneeling and bearing weight through his hands and knees.

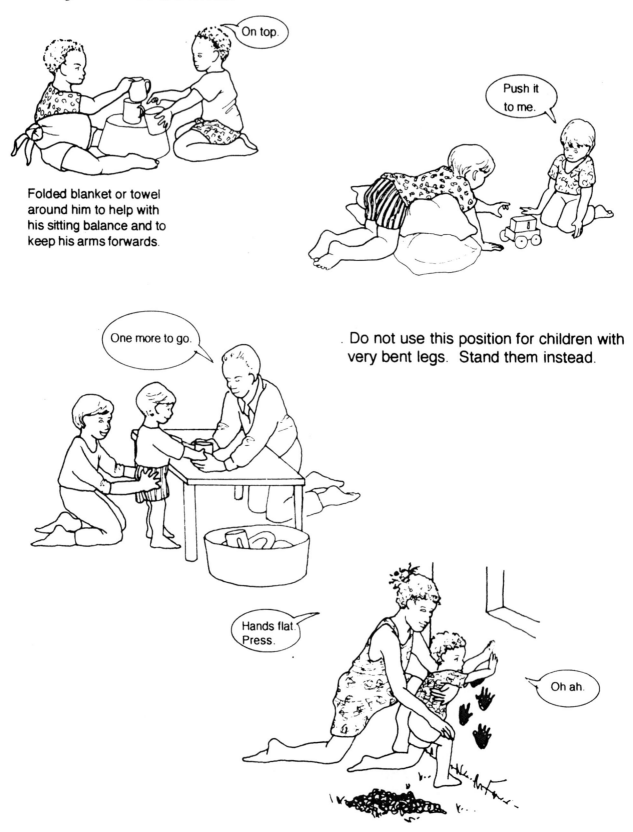

Folded blanket or towel around him to help with his sitting balance and to keep his arms forwards.

. Do not use this position for children with very bent legs. Stand them instead.

62

STAGE THREE

Stage Three: Sitting: <u>Standing Up From a Chair</u>

After she can pull to stand with help, teach her to do it alone. It is often easier for a child with cerebral palsy to stand from a chair, rather than from the floor. Help her to learn the correct movements.

To move from sitting to standing correctly:

. Place her feet flat and underneath her knees.
. She must lean well forward so that her bottom comes off the chair.
. Support her under her arms.
. Practise lifting and lowering her bottom.

Straight knees.

When she can lift her bottom off the chair she is ready to learn to stand.

. As she stands slide your hands down to her elbows, and keep her body forward.
. Stand with straight hips.

Lean forward. Push up.

Then, let her pull herself up.

. If she needs help, press down on her knees as she leans forward to stand.

Stand up. You are nearly straight.

. Now try standing alone.
. If her arms pull back, she should hold a stick to keep them forward.
. Stand with straight hips.

Practise this when washing, dressing, getting off the toilet, and playing.

63

Stage Three: Moving from Place to Place: <u>Squatting and Kneeling Up</u>

Squatting is a good position for stretching tight heels. Many children will need support to balance when squatting. It is important for toiletting and play.

To train squatting:

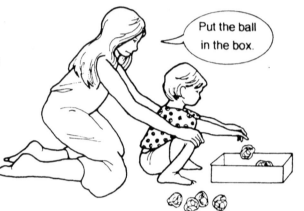

. Help him to balance on his hands and feet.
. Hold his knees.
. Rock him gently in all directions.
. Encourage him to lift one hand up, then the other.

. Push down on his knees while he reaches forward.
. Keep his feet flat.
. Rock him gently in all directions.

. Encourage him to stand from squatting.

> Put the ball in the box.

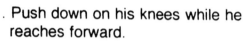

Good kneeling balance makes it easier to stand. To improve kneeling balance:

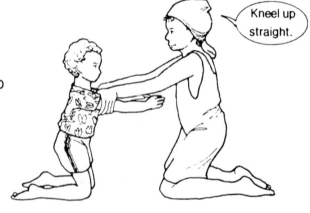

. Start with him sitting on his heels.
. Hold him around his shoulders.
. Help him to lean forward and kneel up until his hips are straight.
. Then help him sit on his heels again.
. Do this slowly.

> Kneel up straight.

. When he is kneeling up push gently from side to side.

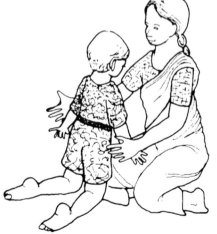

Practise this when washing, dressing, standing from the toilet and playing.

Stage Three: Moving from Place to Place: <u>Walking</u>

To take a step she needs to put her weight on one foot while she lifts the other. Many children will take a long time to learn to walk alone. They may need the help of splints or equipment.

First encourage her to step sideways.

Then encourage her to step forward.

. Support her against your leg and help her to shift her weight from one foot to the other.

As she improves,

. Support her by holding her hips or her elbows.
. Help her to shift her weight to take steps.
. Gradually give less support.

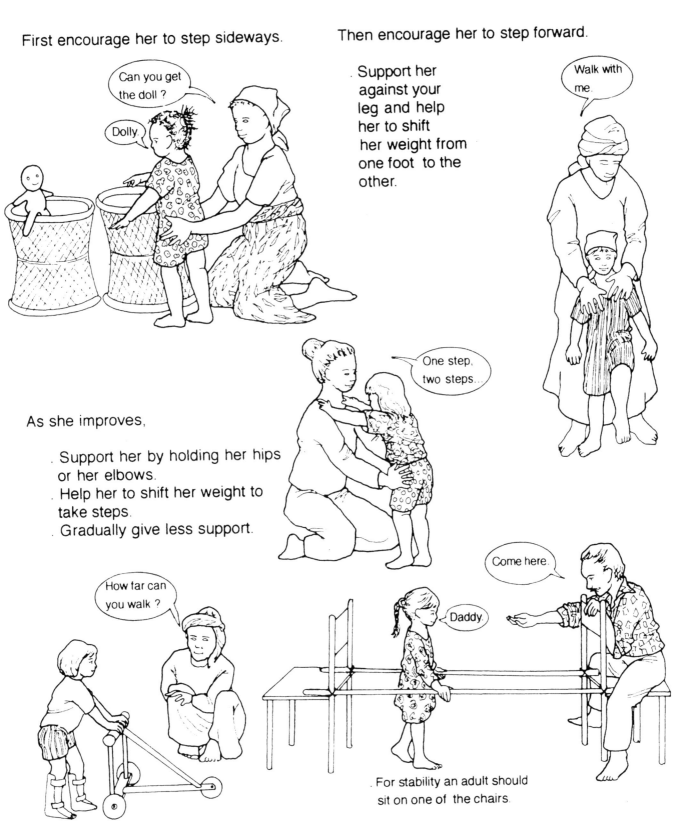

. For stability an adult should sit on one of the chairs.

Practise walking when playing and doing self-care activities.

Stage Three: Self Care: <u>Eating and Drinking</u>

Reduce the support given when eating and drinking, but maintain a good sitting position (see pages 36 to 38). Teach the child to feed himself and to hold a cup. He may still need help to hold his jaw closed (see page 59). Always offer food and drink from straight in front so that he can keep his head forward.

When eating:

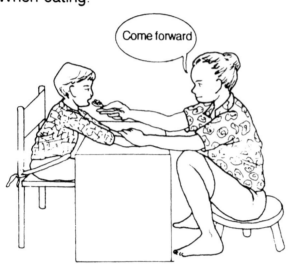

. Help him keep both arms forward with his hands flat on the table while being fed.
. His feet should be flat on the floor.

. Help him to hold the spoon by bending his wrist back.
. Help him keep the other arm forward with his hand flat on the table.
. Use a shallow spoon which will not break easily.

When drinking:

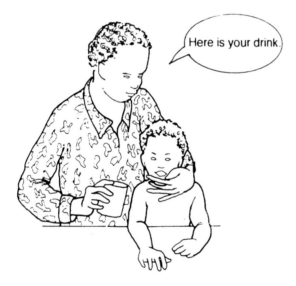

. Keep his arms forward.

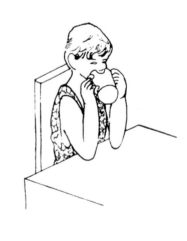

. He holds the cup with both hands and leans on his elbows.

If a child is very floppy and tends to fall forward, use a higher table to support him in a more upright position.

66

Stage Three: Self Care: <u>Washing</u>

Teach the child to start to wash herself. Choose positions which will encourage her to practise sitting and standing. She can learn to wash herself more easily when sitting as this is a more stable position.

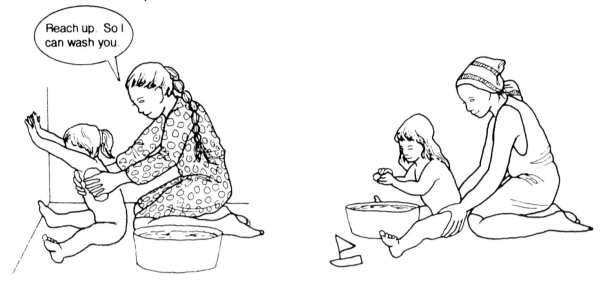

These positions are used to stretch her legs.

If she cannot straighten her knees, she should sit on a stool or a low chair.

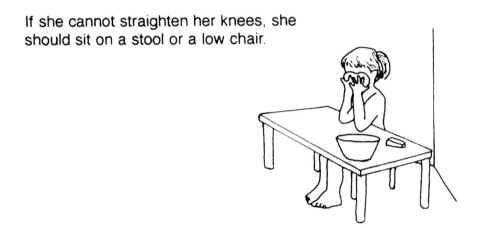

If she is learning to stand, wash her in this position.

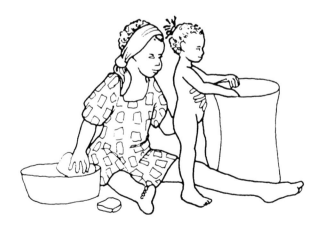

Stage Three: Self Care: <u>Dressing</u>

Teach the child to help when being dressed. Encourage him to lift his arms and legs, or to pull clothes on or off.

Choose positions which will encourage him to practise sitting, kneeling and standing.

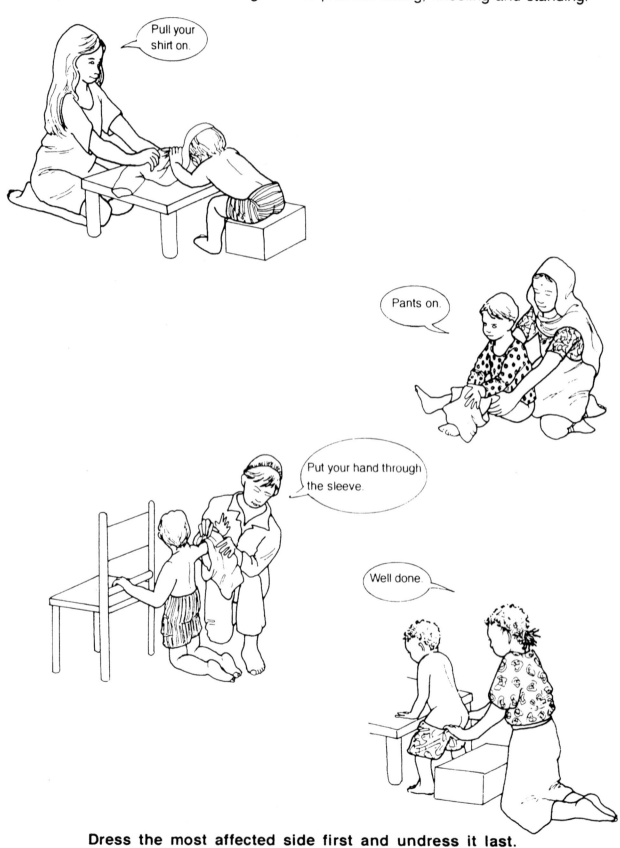

Dress the most affected side first and undress it last.

Stage Three: Self Care: <u>Toiletting</u>

Do not start toilet training until the child is about 18 months old.

Before starting to toilet train a child it is important that you begin to notice when she is peeing and pooing during the day. Keep a record of these times over a few days.

When you have worked out her routine, then you can sit her on a potty at those times each day. If she pees or poos in the potty then praise her. If she does nothing do not scold her but do not praise her either. This will show her that you want her to pee or poo in the potty.

You should not leave her on the potty for more than ten minutes. At first you may have to stay with her. Explain to her what you want her to do.

Eventually she will start to indicate in some way when she wants to go to the toilet. She will still need help to undress and clean herself. She may need help to balance. She may need a special chair so she can sit in a good position.

Some children may not learn to use the potty.

First, support her between your legs.

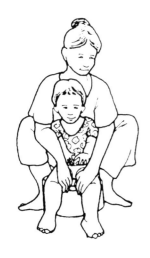
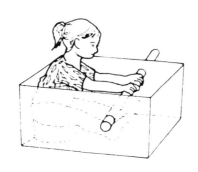
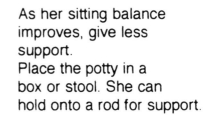

As her sitting balance improves, give less support.
Place the potty in a box or stool. She can hold onto a rod for support.

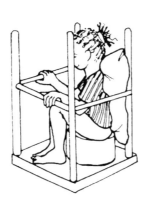

Encourage her to stand from squatting over the toilet.

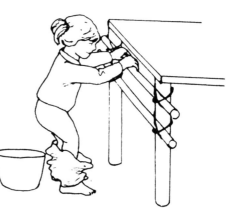

Stage Three: Using Hands and Playing

Encourage the child to move both his arms together and separately. He needs to learn to hold toys and to release them. Play in sitting, kneeling and standing positions.

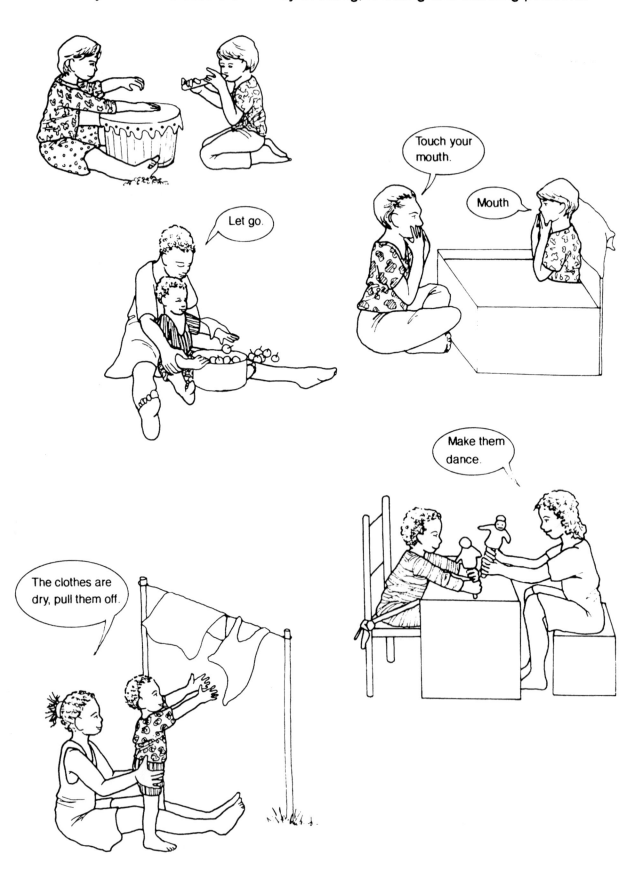

STAGE FOUR

Stage Four: Moving from Place to Place: <u>Walking</u>

Help the child to walk more steadily by further improving her balance. She will also need to learn to step up and down. Walking aids may be needed. Splints may be necessary to hold the feet flat (see page 43).

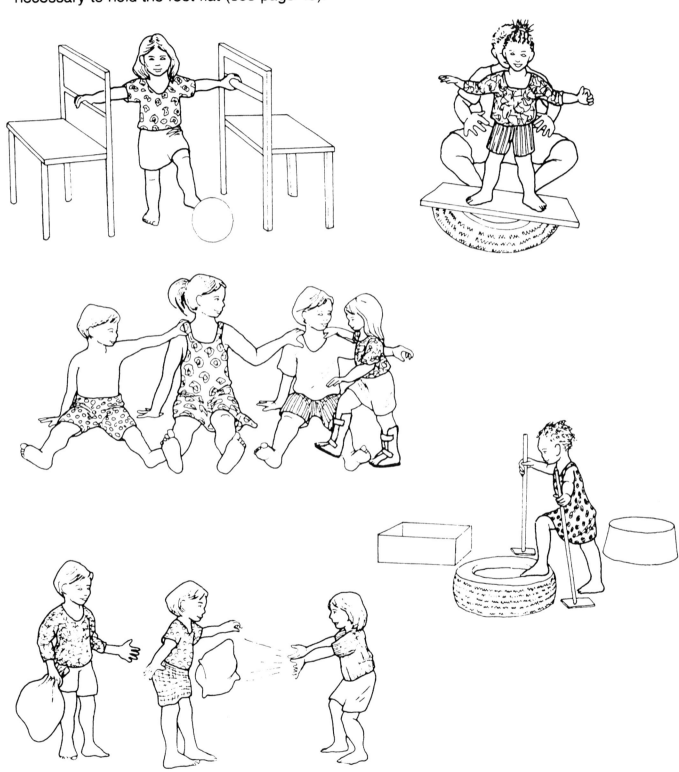

Practise walking when playing and doing self-care activities.

Stage Four: Self Care: <u>Eating and Drinking</u>

If the child has learnt to feed himself, he may need to hold a rod attached to the table to stop his arm pulling back. He should be able to sit in a good position alone or in a chair or on a stool.

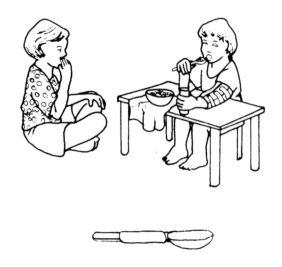

A damp towel or cloth under the plate will stop it from slipping on the table.

The gaiter keeps his arm straight. Holding the rod helps him to keep his arm forward.

He may need to use a spoon with a thick handle to make it easier to hold. Use bamboo, rubber tyre inner tubes or cloth to make a spoon thicker.

Stage Four: Self Care: <u>Washing</u>

If he has learnt to wash himself, he may need to hold onto things for support. He should wash himself in sitting and standing.

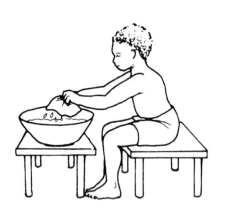
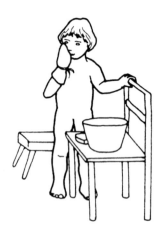

. A soap mitten makes it easier to wash. It is like a glove made from a piece of towel.

Stage Four: Self Care: Dressing

If she has learnt to dress herself she may need to hold onto things or lean against a wall for support. She should dress in lying, sitting or kneeling. Choose the position in which she finds it easiest to do most of it herself.

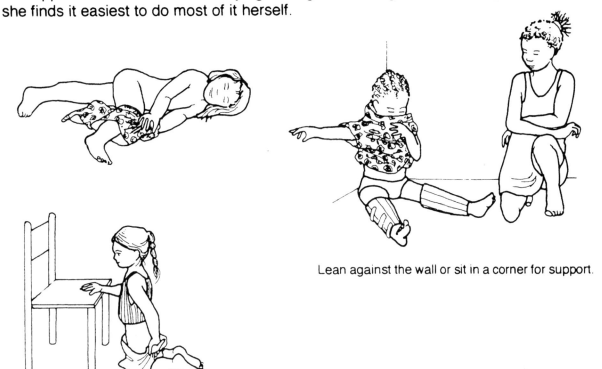

Lean against the wall or sit in a corner for support.

Dress the most affected side first and undress it last.

Stage Four: Self Care: Toiletting

As the child's sitting balance improves, give her less support. Encourage her to help as much as possible with undressing and dressing when going to the toilet. If she can move onto and off the potty or latrine she should be encouraged to do this too.

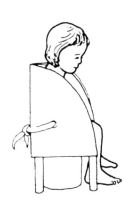

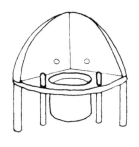

Rods are used to keep legs apart.

A pear shaped seat hole is better for boys.

If squatting balance is poor, give her a stick to hold and a wooden wedge or two bricks to sit on.

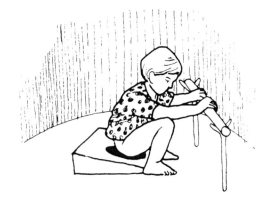

Stage Four: Using Hands and Playing

Encourage the child to play in many different positions. He should open and close his hands and be able to pick up smaller things. Try to encourage him to help in the house. He may still need equipment for support.

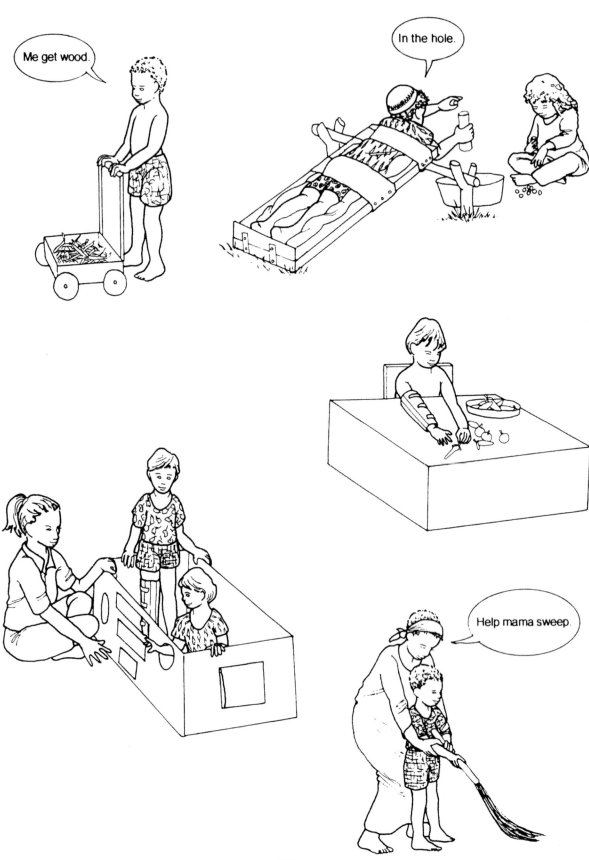

8. TAKING ACCOUNT OF THE PROBLEMS FOUND WITH CEREBRAL PALSY

Very poor eyesight

If by three months a child does not follow a moving light or does not reach out for things, see a doctor for an eyesight test. Very poor sight slows down further the development of movement and learning.

Encourage her to use whatever sight she has.

See "WHO Training Package 1 and 2"

Training suggestions

Lifting
. She may startle and stiffen if she does not see you coming. Prevent this by touching and talking to her first.

Movement
. Let her feel movement. Hold her in a good position and swing or tilt her to increase her confidence. Start by moving slowly.
. Encourage her to explore the floor by rolling and by feeling all around when sitting.
. Encourage her to catch herself when pushed in sitting (see page 55). This takes longer to learn if there is poor sight.

Use of hands
. Guide her arms and hands (see page 32). Encourage her to explore her mother's face and her own body. Touch a toy to the back of her hand. Wait for her to find it and take hold.

Make things easier to see
. Bring the object closer or take her nearer to it.
. Choose a larger toy.
. Choose a bright or shiny toy.
. Make sure the toy moves slowly so she can follow it.

Play with things which are fun to touch and smell.

Difficulties with hearing
. Help her to understand you better when you speak.
. Touch her face to get her attention.
. Stand in front of her with the light on your face.
. Speak loudly and clearly without shouting.
. Use words and gestures at the same time.
. Position her so she can concentrate on listening.

See "WHO Training Package 4 and 5"

Children with Severe Difficulties

Deformities develop most often in the child whose whole body is affected, who moves very little and who also has other difficulties, for example with seeing or learning. A common deformity which occurs is a **windswept deformity**. It occurs when:

The child turns his head to one side only. If the child's head is turned to the right, his knees will also fall to the right. One knee will appear to be further forward than the other because the hips are twisted.

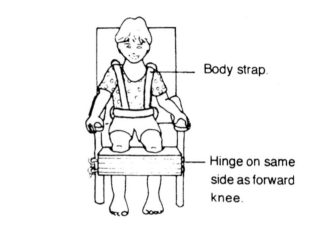

Arm on face side is straight.

Bent arm.

Forward knee.

Hinge.

Knee block.

Sitting:

If the child has very poor balance and keeps sliding out of the chair, try a knee block which will correct his hips and knees. The child may also gain better control of his head and hands.

Make the knee block out of layers of cardboard glued together and padded with cloth or foam.

Only try this if his position can be gently corrected and he can sit comfortably.

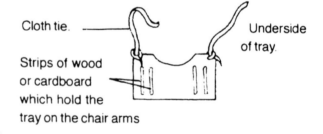

Body strap.

Hinge on same side as forward knee.

He will need a tray to support the body and for toys. Body straps may also be needed. Make holes in the back of the chair for the straps.

Cloth tie.

Underside of tray.

Strips of wood or cardboard which hold the tray on the chair arms

Side Lying:

For some children side lying will be more comfortable. If a child cannot stay on his side, support him with a side lying board. If his legs press together strongly, use a padded wood or cardboard leg shelf to part the legs and prevent pressure on the bottom leg.

Encourage the family to lay him on both sides, if possible, and not just on the side to which he turns his head.

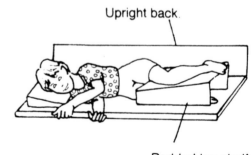

Upright back.

Padded leg shelf.

The best way to prevent deformities, or to slow down their progress, is to put him in a variety of good positions throughout the day.

9. SUMMARY OF WHEN TO ASK FOR MORE HELP

The MLRW should ask for help if:

1. The child shows these early signs of cerebral palsy.

. He feels stiff or floppy most of the time (see page 15).
. Development is slower than expected (see page 15).
. His movements look different from those of other children (see page 16).

To be sure the child has cerebral palsy, refer him to an occupational therapist, physiotherapist, or a doctor.

2. The child has one or more of these problems found with cerebral palsy.

. He has difficulty seeing, he does not follow moving objects by three months of age (see page 75).
. He has a squint after six months of age (see page 7).
. He has difficulty hearing, he does not turn to his own name by six months of age (see page 7 and 75).
. He has fits (see page 8).

Refer him to a primary health care worker for an eyesight or hearing test.

If an eyesight or hearing difficulty is confirmed, the PHCW may refer the child to a doctor. The MLRW should ensure that the family follow up any recommendations made by the PHCW and the doctor.

Take the child to a doctor for advice on medicine to control his fits.

3. Progress with training the child is poor

. The training goals may be too difficult (see page 17).
. He may be too severely affected to progress quickly (see page 17).
. His family may be unable to carry out the training (see page 17).

Take him to a therapist for advice on training goals and what to expect of the child.

Discuss the family situation with the community leaders. Arrange for the community to help support the family.

4. Contractures are getting worse

Active movement, good positioning and passive stretching have been carried out, but the contractures are getting worse (see page 40 and 41).

Take him to a therapist. Plasters, braces or advice about positioning equipment may be needed.

FURTHER READING

The Community Health Worker.
World Health Organisation, 1987 (to be re-issued in 1993).
Distribution and sales, 1211 Geneva 27, Switzerland.

The Education of Mid-Level Rehabilitation Workers.
World Health Organisation, 1992.
Rehabilitation HQ, WHO, 1211 Geneva 27, Switzerland.

Finnie N. (1974)
Handling the Young Cerebral Palsied Child at Home (2nd Ed.)
Butterworth Heinemann Ltd., Linacre House, Jordan Hill, Oxford, OX2 8DP,
England.

Helander E, Mendis P, Nelson G, Goerdt A. (1989)
Training in the Community for People with Disabilities.
World Health Organisation, Distribution and sales, 1211 Geneva 27, Switzerland.

The following Training Packages are referred to in this manual:

For Family Members of People Who Have Difficulty Seeing - 1 & 2.
For Family Members of People Who Have Difficulty Speaking and Hearing
or Speaking and Moving - 4, 5 & 7.
For Family Members of People Who Have Difficulty Moving - 8, 9 & 14.
For Family Members of People Who have Fits - 21.
For Family Members of People Who Have Difficulty Learning - 23.
Breast Feeding a Baby Who Has a Disability - 25.
Play Activities for a Child Who Has a Disability - 26.

Levitt S. (1987)
We Can Play and Move.
Appropriate Health Resources and Technologies Action Group,
1 London Bridge Street, London, SE1 9SG, England.

Packer B. (1986)
IRED Series VI Tools for Africa: Appropriate Paper-based Technology.
IRED East and Southern Africa Office, Box 8242, Harare, Zimbabwe.

Werner D, (1987)
Disabled Village Children.
The Hesperian Foundation, P.O. Box 1692, Palo Alto, California, USA, 94302.

Wirtz S, Winyard S. (1993)
Hearing and Communication for Community Based Rehabilitation Workers.
MacMillan: Teaching Aids at Low Cost, P.O. Box 49, St. Albans, Herts, AL1 4AX,
England.

Acknowledgement

The chart on page 16 is adapted from a leaflet for parents:
    "If You See Any of These Warning Signs".
    Published by: Pathways Awareness Foundation, 123 North Wacker Drive,
    Chicago, Illinois, USA, 60606.